Care of the OSTOMY PATIENT

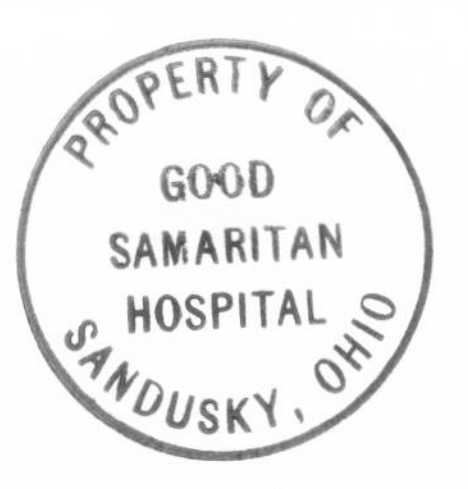

CONTRIBUTORS

ROBERT T. BLAKE, M.D.
Founder of Mission Ostomy Club

LILLIAN FRYE, R.N.
Night Supervisor, Nursing Services

JOHN G. McGREGOR, Jr., M.D.
Gastroenterologist

ALFRED E. STILLMAN, M.D.
Gastroenterologist

DUNCAN CAMPBELL, M.D.
Surgeon

DARWIN W. NEUBAUER, M.D.
Surgeon

PETER C. CROWE, M.D.
Surgeon

HAROLD G. CARSTENSEN, M.D.
Obstetrician and Gynecologist

DONALD GLEASON, M.D.
Urologist

JEAN N. FAULKNER, R.D.
Administrative Dietitian

JACQUELINE R. WOMBLE, B.S., R.Ph.
Adjunct Instructor, College of Pharmacy, and Clinical Pharmacist, University of Arizona

PAMELA MAYHALL, B.S.
Instructor, Human Resources Division, Pima Community College

Care of the OSTOMY PATIENT

VIRGINIA C. VUKOVICH, R.N., E.T.

Ostomy Nurse Clinician, Tucson Medical Center,
Tucson, Arizona

REBA DOUGLASS GRUBB, B.S.

Medical Writer and Education Coordinator,
Instructional Materials, Tucson Medical Center,
Tucson, Arizona; Member, American Medical
Writers Association; Member, National League
of American Pen Women

SECOND EDITION

with 23 illustrations;
drawings by Travis L. Mayhall

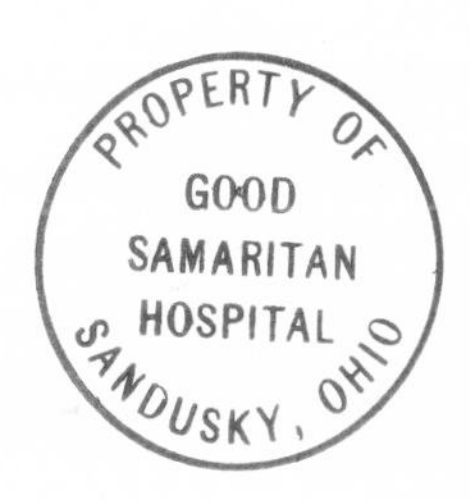

The C. V. Mosby Company

Saint Louis 1977

SECOND EDITION

Previous edition copyrighted 1973

Printed in the United States of America

Distributed in Great Britain by Henry Kimpton, London

The C. V. Mosby Company
11830 Westline Industrial Drive, St. Louis, Missouri 63141

Library of Congress Cataloging in Publication Data

Vukovich, Virginia C 1919-
Care of the ostomy patient.

Bibliography: p.
Includes index.
1. Enterostomy. 2. Surgical nursing. I. Grubb, Reba D., joint author. II. Title. [DNLM: 1. Colostomy. 2. Ileostomy. WI480 V989c]
RD540.V84 1977 617'.43 76-58498
ISBN 0-8016-5276-6

GW/M/M 9 8 7 6 5 4 3 2 1

To progressive practitioners
who become involved with the ostomy patient
and who care enough to accept a new idea
as needs become identified.
Especially do I thank
Dr. Neubauer, Dr. Yoeman, and Dr. Blake,
who stimulated my total commitment
to the ostomy service.

Virginia C. Vukovich

To close associates in the field of nursing
who have inspired and encouraged me
to emit through writing
what I cannot contribute through personal service.
I am especially grateful to nursing professionals,
Lillian Frye, Marjory Olson, Jane Mueller,
and Christine Mahar; and to
Martha Chrisman.

Reba Douglass Grubb

Foreword

The need for ostomy information has existed for a long time. This became manifest after an ostomy department was conceived and developed as an added dimension of patient care through nursing services at Tucson Medical Center.

As for all good advances, inspired and competent leadership was the key ingredient. Mrs. Virginia Vukovich, Tucson Medical Center Ostomy Nurse Clinician, pioneered new levels of patient and physician confidence. The mushrooming interest and desire for more information from patients and staff alike provided a happy alliance of effort with Mrs. Reba Grubb, an accomplished writer and education coordinator at Tucson Medical Center, to produce this book—expanding and presenting a fourfold involvement: physician, patient, family, and nursing staff.

Although we realize that ostomy surgery and the patient's subsequent care is still evolving, this carefully researched treatise throws a practical light on what is now being done to provide better patient care. The "how-to" approach focuses on the patient during presurgical and postsurgical care and throughout social and vocational rehabilitation. The book, in its presentation of basic concepts, will be constructive to the ostomy population, hospital personnel, and associated health colleagues. It will be especially helpful in assisting those without the services of the scarce ostomy nurse specialist, since it offers a step toward individual plans for each patient.

Tucson Medical Center takes pride in the quality of its people's concern for those whom we serve. Mrs. Vukovich and Mrs. Grubb enhance our commitment by their knowledgeable contributions herein.

Donald G. Shropshire

Administrator
Tucson Medical Center
Tucson, Arizona

Preface

The primary objective of this book is to acquaint hospital personnel, students, and other interested persons with the needs of the ostomy patient. It is hoped that, through this knowledge, service to these specific patients will support them in their mental approach to rearranged bodies, enable them to return quickly to normal activities through a procedure of self-care, or, in cases in which patients do not return to health, relieve their pain and discomfort and allow them to die with dignity.

Beginning with the normal digestive tract, we show progressively how the body can develop problems leading to ostomy surgery. Preliminary diagnosis, tests, and resulting surgeries are discussed. Chapters on nutrition, medications, and appliances are offered to acquaint patients and professionals with available products and diets that may best suit the individual. Mention of specific products and name brands should not be construed as exclusive endorsement of those products. Informative chapters on counseling and care of the dying patient will be especially helpful in meeting the patients' emotional needs. Procedures in a step-by-step format simplify methods of hospital patient care and may be adapted to a home nursing care plan. Hospital and community resources to support patients in the hospital, at home, and in the community are also discussed.

Hopefully, through detailed instructions and explanations, this book will communicate to the hospital staff that ostomy surgery carries no more stigma than do other comparable major surgeries. Through understanding and knowledge the staff can effectively counsel and care for patients, allay their fears, and teach them to cope with the many emotional problems of learning to live with appliances for the rest of their lives.

Ostomy as a recognized field is still in its pioneering stages, and information continues to be in short supply although the problem is ancient. Changes in methods of caring for these special patients are emerging. As the ostomy field continues to expand, educational programs nationwide are preparing nurses for this progressive nursing specialty. Educators will find *Care of the Ostomy Patient* valuable as a text or reference.

It is not possible for this text to be all-inclusive regarding the subject of ostomy. It is hoped that you will continue to update your own information and seek out current supportive medical reference books and journals.

We are indebted to the many friends and colleagues who have offered helpful comments, criticisms, suggestions, and contributions. We also wish to extend our gratitude to the individuals from many disciplines who offered information drawn from their practical experience.

We are most grateful to Donald G. Shropshire, Administrator of Tucson Medical Center, for his encouragement; to Orpha Berrie, R.N., Head Nurse, Isolation Unit, Tucson Medical Center; to Lynn Gilbert, Physician's Assistant; to the Education Department of Tucson Medical Center and its staff, Jerry Freund, Director; Tom Krug, Assistant Director; Geraldine Ondov, Jane Mueller, Tina Foote, Education Coordinators; and Jean Good, Office Manager; and to Travis L. Mayhall, artist and draftsman, for his excellent drawings.

Virginia C. Vukovich
Reba Douglass Grubb

Contents

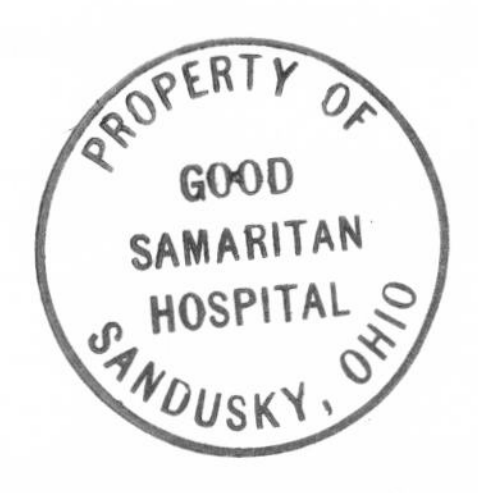

Care of the OSTOMY PATIENT

CHAPTER 1

History

Although diseases of the digestive system are as old as mankind, early treatment was uncertain and often hazardous. Through the persistent and often courageous efforts of medical pioneers, ostomy surgery developed slowly and laboriously, taking centuries to reach its present sophistication.

Early surgery was usually performed for treatment of wounds, abscesses, and amputations because physicians were unable to see inside the human body and could treat only external ailments. The practical anatomic knowledge of the physician was extremely limited. The anatomy of the digestive tract, especially of the abdomen, was beyond the range of his understanding. Obstructions of the digestive tract presented constant problems to the ancients as they still do to modern man because man insists on breaking the natural laws of the mechanism of the human body by overindulgence or eating an inappropriate diet.

Veterinarians were the first to attempt abdominal surgery. Man could not exist without his animals for food and transportation and their care was often more important to him than that of his family. In ancient Thessaly, the land of horses, the public veterinarian was in more demand than the physician. For centuries, veterinarians had successfully treated animals and were skilled in relieving their distended abdomens through puncturing; yet when physicians attempted the same method for human abdominal problems, the results were disastrous.

One of the earliest surgeries on the abdomen occurred in 300 B.C.; it is recorded by Aurelianus Caelius that Praxagoras treated ileus by opening the abdomen, incising the bowel to evacuate it, and then closing it again.

Early surgeries were largely guesswork. Much insight into internal organs was gained in biblical times when diseased or injured animals were slaughtered to determine whether the animal was *kosher* (fit and clean). Herophilus, a pupil of Praxagoras, gained his knowledge as an anatomist by dissection of the human body, and he is known as the contributor of the name "duodenum."

Actually, artists, not physicians, led the way in studying the human body through dissection. They used this method of study in order to correctly draw

☐ From the history collection of Reba Grubb.

the features of what they considered to be the most perfect creation: the human body. From the beginning of the fourteenth century, demonstrations of dissection were held in Bologna, but the physician was still limited in his knowledge of disease because the bodies offered for study were usually young, healthy, executed criminals.

In the Middle Ages, because of belief in the sanctity of the body, this form of study was denied by papal decree. This ban continued until the Renaissance transformed both life and thinking; physicians could then again perform autopsies.

With little knowledge of disease of the abdomen, "passio iliaca" was a popular diagnosis of any disease of the right or left lower abdomen. John of Arderne, Army Surgeon in the Hundred Years War and one of England's earliest surgeons, wrote a treatise on passio iliaca in 1370. Jean Fernel, Professor of Medicine in Paris, wrote in 1567 of a right-side iliac passion. This is believed to have been the first diagnosis of our modern-day appendicitis. Treatment of this disease consisted of draining the abscess. It was not until 1880 that the practice of removing the abscessed appendix was begun by Lawson Tait.

In early medical history, barber surgeons and stone cutters, or lithomists, performed operations. Although the lithomists were noted for the operation of removing kidney stones, their expert help was also required for removal of foreign objects. There is a record that in 1635 a lithomist named Swabe operated on a peasant who had swallowed a knife. The foreign object was carefully positioned inside the abdomen by a magnet; then the lithomist opened the abdomen and removed the knife.

Early physicians were not limited by specialization. Although urology is said to be the oldest surgical specialty, there were few specialists in other surgical fields up to the nineteenth century.

Opening the abdominal cavity had been considered by early surgeons; they had even tried to bring the bowel to the surface. Alexis Littré, surgeon and anatomist of Paris who is known as the "father of colostomy," performed an autopsy in 1710 on a 6-day-old infant who had been born with a malformation of the rectum. He discovered that it was possible to make an incision in the abdomen and either open the two ends of the closed bowel and sew them together or bring the bowel to the surface of the abdomen where it could remain a permanent abdominal anus. Although there is no record that he performed this surgery, his idea was used by several surgeons.

The first successful left iliac colostomy was performed in 1793 by C. Duret, Professor of Surgery at the Military and Marine Hospital of Brest, on a 3-day-old infant born with an imperforate anus. The patient lived to age 45. Seven years later, Professor Fine, Surgeon-in-Chief to the hospital in Geneva, performed the first transverse colostomy on a 63-year-old woman with cancer of the rectum. The patient lived only 3 months, but her death was from the disease, not the operation.

In an attempt to learn more about disease inside the living human body, exploratory laparotomy was advocated but seldom performed. Surgeons were reluctant to open the abdomen for fear that they would not find the disease for which they were looking, thereby subjecting themselves to ridicule. A breakthrough came in 1887 when C. B. Ball of Dublin recommended abdominal colostomy after an exploratory laparotomy of the abdomen. Later, the midline incision was used by Ernest Biles to explore the abdomen, and it became the forerunner of modern exploratory laparotomy methods.

Operations on the small bowel were rare. Although early surgeons believed that ileostomy could be performed, they seldom attempted it. Workable stomas and containers for collecting the dumpings had not yet been designed. Even in the early 1930s it was still an unusual procedure. The incidence of infection in new stomas was high until Rupert Turnbull, a surgeon in Cleveland, Ohio, developed the eversion technique. Later, Bryan Brooke improved upon Dr. Turnbull's idea and perfected the method commonly used today.

Without anesthesia and antiseptics, shock or infection usually resulted from the operation and the patient died. Soldiers with gunshot or sword wounds of the stomach often died from infection. Fecal fistulas that formed in some of the wounds required years to heal. The use of antiseptics and anesthesia, which began in the late nineteenth century, reduced the surgical risk of abdominal operations, and slowly ostomy surgery progressed.

An early operation on the human stomach was the gastrostomy for esophageal cancer, performed by Sedillot in 1846. Operations for pyloric obstructions were usually delayed because of the danger of the operation; surgeons used gastrostomy as a palliative measure only. Gastroenterostomy was later a surgical treatment for gastric ulcers and used as a surgical procedure for peptic ulcers.

Little, if any, progress was made in ostomy surgery of the upper digestive tract until Theodor Billroth, Professor of Surgery at Zurich and Vienna and known as the surgeon of the alimentary tract, performed the first resection of the esophagus in 1872, the first excision of the larynx in 1873, and the first resection of the pylorus for cancer in 1881.

Tracheotomy was performed for croup in 1825 by Pierre Bretomeau. His pupil, French physician Armand Trousseau, pioneered in intubation. An American physician, Joseph P. O'Dwyer, developed a method, often used for diphtheria, to open the larynx at the first sign of suffocation and insert a tube (intubation) so that air could enter the lungs.

During the later years of the nineteenth century, clinical and pathologic descriptions advanced the knowledge of the human body and its many possible deviations from normal healthy digestive processes. Detailed case histories dealing with abdominal diagnoses and surgical procedures were found to be invaluable in the study of medicine. Education in the classroom as well as in the operating room proved to be the prime factor in producing well-trained physicians and surgeons.

Ostomy surgery has now progressed to a special field, not only in surgery but also in the care of the ostomy patient. New methods grow from old ones, and basic to them all is the welfare of the patient, as proved by the thousands of successful ostomy surgeries yearly.

CHAPTER 2

Functions of the ostomy nurse

With the sophistication of surgical techniques, the ostomy field has rapidly expanded so that there are approximately 100,000 new ostomy patients in the United States annually. The complexities of ostomy care, a constant nightmare, produce feelings of inadequacy in the nursing staff, and these emotions are silently communicated to the already disturbed patient. The patient's own emotional trauma, resulting from the now exposed private function and his insecurities regarding the future, builds up, with fears mounting at times to suicidal levels. Psychologically the patient needs to be convinced that his pattern of daily living can be reestablished.

A group of resourceful people, the United Ostomy Association, Inc., and the International Association for Enterostomal Therapists (IAET), had the courage to cope realistically with these problems. They translated concern into a plan of action by establishing special training schools. These schools now produce skilled, efficient enterostomal therapists.

The word "therapist" is often misleading to the laity, who associate the term with medical technicians. The origin of the word is from the Greek *therapeutes,* meaning one who attends the sick. Medical dictionaries define therapist as "a person skilled in the treatment of disease; often combined with a term indicating the specific type of disorder treated."

Enterostomal therapists are specialists who possess the knowledge, training, and ability to care for the ostomy patient. Registered nurses who have a comprehensive knowledge of hospital procedure in the care of the critically ill patient, a general knowledge of drugs, and a positive commitment to aid and instruct the ostomy patient qualify for enterostomal education. It is not uncommon for nurses who are ostomates to enter the ostomy specialty. These professionals often find it easy to establish empathy with the ostomy patient.

Although enterostomy surgeries are more numerous than others, ostomies such as esophagostomy, gastrostomy, tracheostomy, and laryngostomy also have special needs. To care for all ostomy patients, additional education is required. A nurse with this expertise is referred to as a nurse clinician.

The primary goal of the ostomy nurse is to enable patients to leave the hospital with mental and physical confidence in their ability to deal with the changes in body function. As patients recuperate they are supported by the ostomy nurse's knowledge as to management and care of the body, and they plan for normal activities in the future.

Certainly, ostomy patients can survive without the ostomy nurse, but the goal of those who care for the ostomate is adjustment of the patient beyond survival. The patient's rehabilitation will be expedited, his stay in the hospital shortened, and the necessity for possible readmission to the hospital lessened if a satisfactory educational regimen has been given to him. The ostomy nurse has truly opened the door to better ostomy care, which offers the patient an opportunity to live, not merely exist.

The ostomy nurse has five major functions:

1. To assess ostomy patients' needs and ensure that they have a continuity of good care
2. To initiate patient teaching
3. To establish an understanding or liaison with the nursing staff and to aid them in formulating nursing care plans
4. To maintain an adequate recording system
5. To provide an extension of the nurse's knowledge through educational programs

PATIENT ASSESSMENT*

Nursing assessment of the patient is a collection of specific data about the patient, which may begin prior to the patient's referral to the ostomy nurse. The data are gathered and evaluated in a continuing, orderly process. The patient is the primary source.

Assessment provides a basis of information that enables the nurse to plan nursing actions. Reassessment is made as the patient needs change. Observation, interviewing, counseling sessions, and individual informal contacts with the patient are methods of assessment.

Assessment data includes the following:

1. Socioeconomic status
   a. Age, sex, marital status, family relationships
   b. Occupation, financial status, living arrangements
   c. Religious affiliation
   d. Recreational interests
2. Physiologic status
   a. Sensitiveness, hearing, vision, speech, smell, taste
   b. Mobility status: ambulatory, bed rest, range of motion, handicaps
   c. Respiratory status

---

*From material prepared by Reba Grubb for Tucson Medical Center Ostomy Education.

   d. Circulatory status
   e. Nutritional status
   f. Bowel/bladder status
   g. Skin status
3. Emotional status
   a. State of consciousness
   b. Intellectual abilities
   c. Attention span
   d. Patient's perception of the illness

The ostomy nurse has several tools that may be used to assist in assessing the patient's socioeconomic and physiologic status. These include admission information, x-ray studies, laboratory reports, charts of previous admissions, examination reports, and progress reports.

Assessing emotional reactions is more difficult. The nurse must rely on academic and clinical training, intuition, observation, and experience in the art of communication. Self-evaluation of personal attitudes is important if the nurse is to have good nurse/patient communication. For example, as a nurse are you able to:

1. Accept the fact that dealing with excreta is a natural part of the ostomy patient care process?
2. Maintain an awareness that the patient's temporary condition does not compromise his integrity as a human being?
3. Deal with odor that is a problem to both patient and nurse?
4. Deal with emotional problems of the patient?
5. Cope with technical management of the patient's needs?
6. Maintain an ethical (behavioral integrity) attitude in dealing with the ostomy patient and situations that occur?

Following is the *ostomy nurse assessment guide:*

1. Assess patient's perception of diagnosis and severity of illness.
2. Assess patient's understanding of the surgery as explained to him or her by the physician, the anticipated results, and potential behavioral responses
3. Assess the family's understanding of surgery and their ability to cope
4. Assess patient's coping patterns (the patient may not be able to assess realistically his own coping patterns)
5. Assess patient's habits before surgery
   a. Eating and drinking
   b. Elimination
   c. Bowel regularity
   d. Medications taken daily; occasionally
   e. Exercise and sleeping habits
6. Determine preoperatively
   a. Expected extent of surgery

   b. Type of stoma
   c. Evaluation of stoma site
   d. Expected physical activities after recovery
7. Recognize symptoms of complications
   a. Intake and output
   b. Abnormal odors
   c. Skin abnormalities
   d. Changes in stoma—size, color
   e. Infectious lesions
   f. Obstructions
   g. Wound dehiscence
8. Prepare nursing care plans
9. Assess patient's strengths
   a. Dexterity
   b. Mental acuity
   c. Handicaps
10. Assess patient's reaction to self-care
    a. Exhibited interest
    b. Rejection
    c. Ability to observe
    d. Ability to learn
11. Assess patient's fantasies about the attitude of others
    a. Toward his stoma
    b. Toward dating
    c. Toward marriage
    d. Toward pregnancy
    e. Toward sexual relations
12. Assess patient's attitude toward returning to school or to a vocation
13. Assess patient's attitude toward reassuming hobbies, sports, travel
14. Assess ostomate visitation
    a. When visit should occur
    b. Patient's reaction to the idea of a visit
    c. Patient's reaction to the visit
15. Assess medications
    a. Does patient need a stool softener?
    b. Does patient need a medication to firm or deodorize the stool?
    c. Are medications necessary for flatus problems?
    d. Recognize the hypersensitive patient's need for a tranquilizer or the depressed person's need for a mood elevator, and report this assessment to the physician
16. Assess nutritional needs
    a. Does patient need a bulk producer?
    b. Should the patient continue low residue? Hyperalimentation? Other special diet?

17. Assess patient's need for irrigation
18. Observe need for aid in securing supplies
    a. Financial
    b. Location of supply source

PATIENT TEACHING*

Motivation and patient interest are significant in attaining rehabilitation. The patient and his family should be made aware of the total care approach, which extends from admission to discharge, through transfer to either an extended care facility or home. Teaching is therefore an important function of the ostomy nurse.

Patient teaching is communication that involves the receiving of information from the patient and the giving of information to the patient by the nurse. If the patient is too ill to comprehend a plan of care, the teaching could begin with the family. Information gathered in the patient assessment can be used to support a teaching plan.

Ostomy nurses vary in patient teaching experience, and some may be unprepared to accept this responsibility. Clinicians trained to perform this function may be called in to assist the ostomy nurse.

The following points may be utilized in patient teaching:

1. The teaching plan should be discussed with the physician.
2. The nurse should not become so involved with emphasis on actual procedure that the individual is neglected.
3. All patient teaching should be recorded on the patient's nursing care plan and reviewed at each shift change to modify the teaching plan as necessary.
4. The complete procedure should be presented in steps related to the whole.
5. When guiding the patient toward self-care, it is important to teach the patient the procedure in the way it will be carried out in the home situation. The equipment the patient is to use, or similar equipment, should be employed in teaching.
6. The teaching should occur at the time of day the patient expects to perform the procedure at home and not at the convenience of the hospital personnel.
7. If possible, the ostomy nurse should simulate a homelike atmosphere.
8. Facts should be stated one at a time, and the instructions repeated at intervals until the nurse is satisfied that the patient can perform independently.
9. Interaction with the patient should be informal.

---

*From instructional materials prepared by Reba Grubb for Tucson Medical Center Education Department.

10. Take-home instructions should be provided for the patient. This is positive reenforcement of the teaching process.
11. The patient should not be forced to learn. Repetition is the key to impressing facts on the patient's mind. It is unrealistic to believe that all patients will be able to assume self-care.
12. Wherever possible, teaching should begin within 24 to 36 hours, depending on the patient's progress and alertness.
13. Examples of both positive and negative situations should be presented to the patient.
14. Three or more teaching sessions should be planned. If only one session is possible, select the most meaningful aspects of the procedure and concentrate on the patient's functional abilities to learn.
15. Teaching aids should be used to encourage patient learning. These may include a diagram of the involved anatomy, pictures, pamphlets, graphs, charts, slides, and videotapes.
16. Questions from the patient should be encouraged to promote a better teaching/learning situation.
17. Terminology used in teaching should be matched to the education and understanding level of the patient.
18. Hospital and community resources should be discussed with the patient and emotional support promoted through trained visitors who have had similar experiences.
19. The nurse should make a careful observation of the difficult patient's behavior. Personal feelings of the nurse should be stated in a team conference and the behavior of the patient examined objectively, including the patient's point of view. An approach to the problem should be planned, a realistic goal set, and a specific time for evaluation made.

NURSING CARE PLANS

Uniformly good care in a positive atmosphere is vital to an ostomy patient, who is already having difficulty adjusting to his new body image. Long weekends or periods when the ostomy nurse must be away can prove difficult for the staff and upsetting to the patient if the staff is not familiar with the ostomy program. Nursing care plans may guide the staff in the continuation of this care.

Although the underlying principles of routine patient care are the same, nursing plans for the ostomy patient must be individualized according to his type of surgery, condition, and existing situation. Personalized systematic plans provide an opportunity for the nursing staff to share continuity and communication of the patient's care throughout the 24-hour period. It also enables the staff who are not acquainted with the patient to effect an understanding before they meet. It is the responsibility of the ostomy nurse to plan with the physician, the staff nurse, and usually the family the most beneficial individual patient care pattern.

The concept of planned care focuses on the patient, encourages more effective utilization of the nurse's knowledge, and aids in evaluating the patient's needs and in classifying him according to high, average, or low dependency care. The nurse's plan for the patient may have already been initiated *before* the patient is admitted. The hospital nursing care plan usually begins soon *after* the patient is actually in the hospital.

Data gathering, whether impromptu or carefully designed, is a basic factor in the process of patient care planning. Preliminary plans are formed as the nurse or attendants talk to the patient and observe his appearance, expressions, and behavior. The process develops as the nurse learns the patient's history from him, his family, and his physician. Planning conferences and patient status reporting provide the essential ingredients that elevate the quality of the plan.

The planning conference. The planning conference is designed to explore problems or any situation in which the patient might benefit from the assistance of the nurse and to aid the nurse in arriving at a tentative course of action. It involves team members who serve the area in which the patient is being attended. The number of team members will vary according to patient requirements. Teams usually include the staff nurse, a licensed practical nurse, nurse assistants, students, and resource personnel. Each member of the team will have opportunities for activating the various ingredients of the care plan regardless of the level of responsibility. For example, many pertinent aspects are observed by the nurse assistant who is alert to situations as personal care is administered to the patient.

The following points might be considered in a planning conference:

1. Coordinate all available services by utilizing the ostomy nurse, head nurse, and other resource personnel such as the dietitian, therapists, social worker, clergy, and family.
2. Stress that the conference is concerned with the care of an *individual* and that cooperation is necessary in interpreting his problems.
3. Consider the individual's personality and idiosyncrasies.
4. Explore the meanings of factual data and actual observations.
5. Note the emotional status and reactions of the patient.
6. Use the exchange of information to promote incidental teaching opportunities for patient or staff.
7. Thoroughly discuss what can be done to improve the nursing care.
8. Record the problem and an approach to the solution.

Patient status reporting. A comprehensive pertinent report from one shift to the next is essential. A patient's status affects a nursing care plan. Any unusual occurrence during the previous 8 hours is of consequence to the oncoming nursing personnel. It may be a recording or person-to-person report.

Points in reporting

1. Report in intelligible terms.
2. Emphasize constructive and positive factors.
3. Adhere to objectives and principles of medical/surgical nursing care.
4. Report clear, concise, meaningful information and data.
5. Recount actual observation, not opinion, of the patient's progress and reactions.

Contents of the report

1. Patient's progress within the previous 8 hours
2. Hygiene and physical comfort
3. Activities (exercise, rest, sleep)
4. Safety measures instituted for prevention of accident or injury
5. Any indications of infection
6. Nutrition—patient's response
7. Problems in intake, output, and electrolyte balance
8. Physiologic responses to his condition
9. Positive and negative expressions
10. Any new or revised procedures initiated

Outline of nursing care plans. The topics listed here may serve as a guide toward formalizing the individual care plans. Specific instructions for the patient should be fully explained—for example, the patient's attitude may require a lengthy report, or his skin care may involve a battery of procedures to solve the problem.

Observe and record

1. Patient's attitude: toward his illness, toward his stoma, toward his future
2. Fluid intake and output; electrolyte balance
3. Condition of skin circumostomy
4. Significant changes in patient's condition
5. Any evidence of infection (report to physician)

Hygienic needs

1. Odor management
2. Oral care
3. Aseptic care of nasogastric tubes, catheters, and tracheostomy tubes
4. Disposal of dressings, tissues, cotton balls, and secretions
5. Change of appliance

Irrigation (if necessary)

1. Method
2. Time and results

Comfort measures and emotional support

1. Positioning the patient
2. Patient's preferences of physical environment
3. Body care

4. Additional counseling (planned time in patient's room)
5. Spiritual care

Nutrition

1. Low-residue diet
2. Trial foods
3. Foods to avoid

Medications

1. Precautions
2. Allergies or dermatitis

Patient teaching

1. Familiarization with the word "stoma"
2. Encouragement of patient to help himself: exercises, deep breathing, assisting with appliance change

Specifics relating to laryngostomy or tracheostomy

1. Airway patency
   a. Supporting head while turning or elevating
   b. Frequent suctioning
   c. Cleaning of cannula
2. Observe
   a. Signs of excessive bleeding and drainage
   b. Moisture
   c. Mouth care
3. Communication
   a. Pad and pencil
   b. Illustrations
   c. New speech teaching plans
4. Nutrition
   a. Tube-feeding plan
   b. Variables of tube feeding

Continuity of care

1. Referral to community resources
2. Extended care facility referral
3. Home

Evaluating the nursing care plan. The nursing plan should be evaluated to determine its effectiveness and to help build skills in gathering data, formulating plans, and carrying out the plans for maximum benefit to the patient. There are several methods of evaluating the plan:

1. A nursing audit of the plans and progress notes
2. Follow-up nursing conference
   a. Was the staff satisfied with the care of the patient?
   b. Could the plan have been different?
   c. Should it have included aspects that were not covered?
   d. Were individual needs recognized?

e. Did it cover limitations and strengths of the patient?
f. Did it help to prevent anticipated problems?
g. Were the goals achieved?

3. Observation of the discharged patient through the physician's office or through the specialist's clinical follow-up as to patient's adjustment to normal living
4. The patient's own reaction to his care (This may be accomplished through a printed form that is given to the patient upon discharge, requesting a reaction to his stay in the hospital.)

Nurse audit.* The patient's chart is a communication between the physician and nursing personnel. This written communication must be accurate and adequate for at least two reasons: (1) to provide good personal continuity of care and (2) to legally protect the patient, physician, hospital, and employees.

The purpose of an audit is to evaluate the quality of nursing care that is given to the patient and to determine whether policies of charting are being followed.

Most hospitals have an auditing committee who produce their own guide for establishing professional accountability. The guide consists of the following:

1. Written standards for types of audits and components of patient care
2. An instrument by which to measure each standard
3. Method of implementation

Basically there are two types of nursing audits:

1. *Outcome (closed) audit*—an evaluation of patient charts after the patient has been discharged
2. *Process (open) audit*—an evaluation of patient charts while the patient is still an inpatient

Four components of patient care that should be audited are nursing care Kardex, the Medex, bedside care, and the manner in which the charting is done.

RECORDS AND REPORTS

Record keeping is important in the care of the ostomy patient. The patient's chart is a yardstick to measure his needs and progress, and it should be adequately maintained.

Each institution has specific methods and forms for charting the patient's progress. The two forms shown here pertain to the ostomy nurse's recordings.

Recording ostomy consultation. When services of the ostomy nurse are requested by the physician, pertinent information regarding all aspects of care

---

*From a lecture by Jane Mueller, R.N., Education Coordinator, Tucson Medical Center.

Patient's name
or stencil

Ostomy nurse

Date	Time	
		Ostomy services

Fig. 2-1. Ostomy nurse consultation sheet.

and observations by the nurse should be recorded and become a permanent part of the patient's chart. A standard consulting form may be used by the nurse or a special form may be designed for this purpose (Fig. 2-1).

Ostomy patient record. The ostomy nurse should personally keep a record of each service performed for the ostomy patient. A patient record card serves as a convenient and quick reference when needed (Fig. 2-2).

Annual report. Records are essential to the preparation of the ostomy nurse's annual report to the administration or to the Board of Directors. This report should contain the following:

A. General assessment of the past year
  1. Accomplishments or setbacks
     a. Procedures initiated
     b. Improvements
     c. Problems
     d. Projects
  2. Number of patients attended
     a. Inpatients
     b. Outpatients
        (1) Clinic

Ostomy patient record

Name: ____________ Account No. ____
Address: ____________ Med. Rec. No. ____
Adm. date: ______ Disc. date: ______ D.O.B. ____
Telephone: ______ Doctor: ______
Agency: ______ Diagnosis: ______
Visits or service: ______ Room No. ______

Date	Code No.	Charges	Remarks
1.			
2.			
3.			
4.			
5.			
6.			
7.			
8.			
9.			

Fig. 2-2. Ostomy patient's record card.

(2) Home visits
(3) Other hospitals or extended care facilities visited

3. Classes taught
   a. Number and type of classes
   b. Number and type of students
      (1) Professional
      (2) Nonprofessional
      (3) Related services personnel

B. Continuing education—any learning media attended by the ostomy nurse or specific ostomy personnel
   1. Meetings, seminars, workshops
   2. In-service training courses
   3. College courses

C. Goals
   1. Not accomplished
   2. Future

D. Special expenditures

EDUCATION

The annual increase in ostomy surgeries and the emergence of new techniques and new equipment have, more than any other factors, created a dilemma for practitioners in this field. Recruitment of trained personnel is difficult because of the increased demand for ostomy services and the few comprehensive ostomy training schools available. Physicians realize that the cure of the ostomy patient depends significantly on the continuity of nursing care, and they offer the nursing staff the benefit of their expertise in counseling, training, and guidance. However, physicians are not free to devote the time necessary for producing trained personnel. Therefore the most feasible avenue of effectively coping with this need is through the initiation of new, comprehensive education programs and the updating of existing programs by both hospitals and nursing schools.

Students of ostomy education come from professional and nonprofessional levels, and the content and curricula should be geared to the needs of the participants. Training may help solve immediate problems and also provide a continuing education process.

To complement and extend this educational process, several program options are available, such as orientation, in-service education, new nursing school curricula, workshops, community or regional meetings, opportune teaching, high school health career days, and continuing education. One of these should meet the needs of the student population involved and of the institution or agency offering the course.

Before a specific program is planned, there must be a conceptual knowledge of the total training to be accomplished and the processes of planning required to effectively promote programs.

The planning process. Planning is essential if programs are to be meaningful, functional, and enriching. The following are involved in the planning process:

1. Obtaining the cooperation of the administration and the director of nursing service
2. Selecting a planning committee
3. Determining basic objectives
4. Defining essentials that are required in designing the course
5. Identifying needs
6. Discussing methods and aids of instruction
7. Securing qualified instructor(s)
8. Defining categories of students
9. Scheduling the programs
10. Making physical arrangements
11. Contacting participants
12. Introducing speakers
13. Preparing publicity
14. Outlining the program
15. Evaluating

The planning committee. Members of the committee should be persons with special knowledge selected to fit the program's design. Usually the committee will be composed of the ostomy nurse, director of nursing service, a representative from the medical/surgical staff, and members of related services.

The ostomy nurse usually assumes the responsibility of the program content, goals, and purposes of the course. The details involved in the planning process are executed or delegated by the committee. The complexity of the program dictates the degree of involvement. Frequently the ostomy nurse and the education coordinator assume the responsibility for the program. The education coordinator is valuable in the complicated task of planning. A coordinator is usually available in hospitals through either the supervisory nursing staff or an established education department. This is a resource person with expertise in the education processes to whom the director of nursing service, hospital administration, or the education department delegates the responsibility for the actual administration of the various programs. The coordinator also may be utilized in an advisory capacity only, depending on the ostomy-oriented resource personnel available. Some functions of the coordinator may be:

1. To serve as a consultant
2. To supervise activities of the program
3. To participate in teaching
4. To serve as an evaluator of the program, criticizing performance
5. To aid in physical arrangements and in contacting the speakers
6. To act as liaison between community, hospital, and nursing schools if the program extends beyond the hospital domain
7. To help in the selection of methods and teaching aids
8. To determine needs and resources
9. To serve as arbitrator in the event one is necessary in decision making
10. To research sources
11. To secure trained personnel to operate audiovisual equipment

Objectives. Ostomy education is guided by basic objectives. Underlying these objectives is the philosophy of the ostomy service, which is based on the worth of the individual, the belief that each patient has the right to comprehensive support throughout the span of his illness, and the knowledge that this care will facilitate the patient's restoration to his pattern of life as rapidly as possible in the best state of mental and physical health attainable for him.

Stated objectives reflect the purposes of education and give direction to the individual programs. They also help the teacher envision content, activities, and evaluation methodology. Ostomy education objectives may be stated as follows:

1. To promote the improvement of patient care by improving the competence, performance, and understanding of the personnel
2. To coordinate the total ostomy program of the hospital
3. To assess educational needs of those caring for the ostomy patient
4. To develop sound training programs to meet the needs of the personnel

5. To provide and recommend teaching materials
6. To review and evaluate the programs
7. To motivate personnel to continue their education
8. To identify opportunities for additional study, research, and action concerning the ostomy patient
9. To cooperate with pertinent resource agencies in the promotion and development of stimulating health careers programs
10. To keep informed concerning new developments, new equipment, and new techniques on both the local and the national levels, and to utilize and disseminate such information as is appropriate

Essentials. Essentials to a successful program follow:

1. A realistic identified need
2. Evidence that the need will promote a learning process that can attract sufficient support to create participation
3. The ability to develop a plan of action

Identifying needs. Identification of needs is a major factor in selecting the content and level of a program. Needs include the acquisition or the changing of an attitude or point of view as well as attaining knowledge or skills. There are several approaches available to determining and analyzing needs.

Direct identification. A physician may identify a particular need and ask that a program be initiated to meet it.

Observation. The ostomy nurse may systematically observe personnel as they care for the ostomy patient. The observation should be conducted on all three shifts as to work performance, attitudes, skill and efficiency, technical knowledge employed, and communication. The results of these observations should be analyzed and a priority of needs established.

Personal interviews. A one-to-one interview with personnel who are directly involved with the ostomy patient will frequently afford feedback to the ostomy nurse, identifying the need for a specific training program.

Questionnaire. With the consent of the administrative or departmental supervisors, hospital personnel may be given the opportunity of identifying needs and assisting with program planning through the use of a questionnaire, such as shown on p. 20.

The questionnaire should be tabulated and analyzed. All needs are examined and scheduled for either immediate or long-range programs.

Patient feedback. The ostomy nurse should occasionally attend ostomy club meetings. The opinions expressed by new or established ostomates will reflect the patient's needs and contribute to patient teaching objectives.

Methods. Methods are designed to aid in the presentation of materials, knowledge, concepts, and ideas. Effective utilization of methods will determine to some degree the success or failure of a program; therefore the choice of technique is a matter of some consequence.

Methods are not a cure-all for teaching problems, but they do offer opportunities for improving learning and can promote good teaching when thought-

---

We need your help in determining what you wish to learn about the aspects of ostomy. Answers to the following questions will indicate the need for various topics to be included in an educational program. Please fill in and return to ______________.

Check one: PROFESSIONAL ________ NONPROFESSIONAL ________
Signature is optional.

I am interested in:

1. Ostomy anatomy and physiology
2. Symptoms, diseases, and diagnostic procedures predisposing to ostomy surgery
3. Types of ostomy surgery (Adult ____ Pediatric ____)
   a. Ileostomy, total colectomy
   b. Colostomy, temporary or permanent; double-barrel, loop, sigmoid transverse
   c. Cecostomy
   d. Urinary diversions—ileal conduit, cystostomy, ureterostomy, nephrostomy
4. Counseling patients
5. Preoperative care
6. Postoperative care
7. Skin excoriation
8. Types of appliances and methods of application
9. Fluids and dehydration
10. Diet
11. Medications
12. Resources in the hospital and community; ostomy clubs
13. Nursing care plans, patient conferences, and reports
14. Odor control
15. Improving communication with patients
16. Handling of emergencies
17. Interesting patients in self-care
18. Ostomy terminology

---

fully planned and properly utilized. Methods vary with the subject, instructor, students, time, and resources available. They frequently intermix for more meaningful interpretations.

Lecture. The lecture is an informative address by an expert on a series of related ideas and facts. It offers the student an opportunity for learning through note taking and a question and answer period. All lectures should be followed by an adequate question and answer session.

The modern concept of the lecture is the combination of this method with other methods (for example, demonstrations) and training aids (films, charts, and the like). Lectures should be well rehearsed to assess quality of delivery, length of presentation, time, and organization of content.

Dramatization. Dramatization is a teaching method that may be used to depict any aspect of a given situation. The use of drama provides an opportunity for the student to learn what it may feel like to face a situation that he cannot experience firsthand and to get closer to certain realities. By reconstructing the experience he may relive the emotional experiences of an ostomate trying to learn how to apply a pouch or perform an irrigation. The most effective dramatizations for classroom presentation are usually short prepared skits or improvised role play.

Demonstration. A demonstration is a planned presentation of certain procedures, skills, or products performed by a well-qualified person. It involves "doing" plus "telling," and it can stimulate learning by encouraging the student to practice his own interpretation of the demonstration just performed. Proper preparation is essential to the success of the demonstration; each step should be planned and rehearsed in advance. Time should be allowed for questions so that all points are clearly understood.

Some suggestions for an effective demonstration follow:

1. Demonstrate where all members of the class may see and hear.
2. Demonstrate correctly.
3. Plan well and follow the plan.
4. Explain the steps in simple language.
5. Check periodically for the effectiveness of the demonstration.
6. Review and summarize the main points.
7. Allow time for questions, answers, and practice session.

Case study. The case study is a detailed description of a patient in a situation that represents a problem to be resolved. It should be as complete as possible without the use of unnecessary words. Case studies vary widely in length according to the complexity of the situation.

This method develops analytic skill. It encourages the student to present problems, seek solutions to the problems, learn to analyze them, and participate in discussion. Two methods of selecting situations for this case study may be employed.

1. The instructor may have the option of presenting cases that have proved beneficial and interesting to other students.
2. The student may bring an experienced or researched situation to share with the class.

Here are guidelines for preparing a case study of an ostomy patient*:

Selection of case and collection of data

1. Patient's initial (or name)
2. Diagnosis
3. Pertinent history
   a. Age
   b. Marital status
   c. Family
   d. Race
   e. Religion
   f. Occupation

*From instructional materials prepared by Reba Grubb for Tucson Medical Center Education Department.

Patient profile

1. Nurse assessment
2. Physical findings
   a. Hospital workup
   b. Laboratory findings
   c. Diagnostic tests
   d. Present illness: severity and brief history
   e. Appearance, impressions, handicaps, allergies
3. Emotional status
   a. Patient's understanding of illness, subsequent surgery, and results
   b. Body image
   c. Sexual interest
   d. Reaction of patient to hospital environment
4. Patient's family
   a. Understanding of patient's illness, surgery, and possible change in home routine
   b. Ability to cope
   c. Knowledge and factors that might affect hospital care and future of patient

Preoperative care

1. Counseling the patient
2. Marking stoma site
3. Preparation for diagnostic measures

Surgical procedure

1. Brief description of surgery
2. Patient's condition; any complications

Postoperative care

1. Immediate postoperative assessment
2. Pathologic changes
3. Assessment of
   a. Intake and output; fluids and electrolyte balance
   b. Appearance of stoma; changes in shape or color
   c. Effluent consistency and color
   d. Odor problems
   e. Medications and treatment modalities
   f. Skin care: routine and problems
4. Temporary appliance and accessories
   a. Type and reason for choice
   b. Application and removal
5. Irrigation (if applicable); timing and routine
6. Nutritional considerations: special diets; provision for late evening snack if pre-illness routine included this (For example, the patient may have worked a night shift for several years and established eating habits to accommodate this pattern.)

Nursing action based on patient's need

1. Nursing care plan
   a. Formulation of remedial plan and recommendations
   b. Considerations for continuity in 24-hour care

c. Modifications in care plan as indicated
d. Safety measures
e. Personal hygiene
2. Medical treatment plan
3. Patient teaching
a. Counseling
b. Appliance care
c. Preparation of patient for expectations of change in normal routine
4. Family teaching
5. Description of special care (if given)
6. Interaction with special services
a. Social services
b. Respiratory services
c. Occupational therapy
d. Physical medicine and rehabilitation; body mechanics
7. Counseling sessions on emotional, spiritual, and mental needs of patient

Discharge planning
1. Home routine
2. Vocational or school considerations
3. Social and economic needs
a. Hobbies
b. Sports
c. Travel
d. Church and social activities
e. Financial aid: Medicare, American Cancer Society, Crippled Children's Clinic, others
f. Community resources: Visiting Nurse Association, Public Health Nurse, school nurse, industrial nurse
4. Permanent appliance fitting and information on purchase of supplies
5. Ostomy club visitor
6. Transfer to extended care facility (if indicated)
7. Take-home instructions

Follow-up to determine effectiveness of measures applied
1. Home visits if needed
2. Clinic visits scheduled
3. Regular checkups suggested

Evaluation of study

Summary and comments

Pathology department slides. Pathology department slides are an adjunct in teaching and understanding the cellular changes in the body necessitating ostomy surgeries. The pathologist will be able to make a thorough interpretation of the slides to the class.

Clinical instruction. No method of instruction, however well conceived, can supplant the basic learning medium of bedside teaching. An old Chinese adage supports the psychologic principle that one has a better conception of that which he sees and does than that which he only hears.

When I hear it I forget it
When I see it I remember it
When I do it I know it

Educational activities of the hospital are enriched when students learn in the atmosphere of the subject that they are being taught. When observation is combined with participation it becomes more meaningful.

Clinical teaching brings the classroom to the bedside, where the problems grow more real and interesting as a result of practice. Once the student has accomplished the task himself, he is well on the way to mastering it.

This method points up the fact that each patient is an individual with unique problems, just as each student is unique in learning methods of coping with the patient's problems. Both classroom and clinical teaching increase the student's ability to learn.

Field trips. A field trip is a learning method that links classroom theory to practiced reality. It increases student interest in content by relating classroom experience to functional settings. An ostomy student's attitudes may be influenced by a visit to related services clinics such as Crippled Children's, Cerebral Palsy, Speech, or Cancer Clinics, as well as observations of intramural services.

This method of training requires considerable class time and therefore must be justified in terms of educational gains.

Panel presentation. The panel presentation customarily involves three to six persons selected on the basis of interest in and knowledge of the subject. Verbal skill is also a qualification for both the panel members and the moderator. Although the participants are usually unrehearsed, except for a brief meeting before the presentation to discuss a general method of procedure, they are contracted far in advance of the program to allow ample preparation time.

The most successful panel presentations include a period for audience participation. The panel members are usually seated at a table facing the audience, and they exchange views on a particular topic. The panel is a very flexible method, and the moderator should have expertise in varying the pace of the meeting by making use of opportunities as they are presented.

Teaching materials. Teaching materials can make the learning experience more concrete. New advances in materials are constantly emerging, and catalogs are available for selection. However, many effective teaching materials may be improvised by the teacher, student, speaker, or education department.

The instructor usually selects the materials, since the objective of the course must be considered. Following are a few of the many teaching aids available.

Exhibit. An exhibit is a planned display of related materials that communicate certain ideas and information on a specific topic. The materials may involve audiovisual presentations, products, collections, or illustrations such as line drawings, photographs, or charts. The exhibit is usually placed in the hall, anteroom, or a prominent corner of the auditorium or classroom.

Suggestions for preparing exhibits include the following:

1. Display a message in a glance whenever possible.
2. Place the exhibit where it can best be seen.
3. Present only one idea to an exhibit, or give related ideas in separate sections of the exhibit (for example, appliances for the colostomate and for the ileostomate).
4. Draft legends so that they are brief, simple, uniform, and legible.
5. Use contrast and color.
6. Use motion for more intricate exhibits (turntable, action figures, filmstrips).

Chalkboards. The chalkboard is a well-known tool to teachers. In ostomy training it may be effectively utilized for writing nursing plans, preparing procedures, or listing terminology.

Models. A model may be the ''Mrs. Chase'' doll used in teaching, or it may be a recognizable imitation of the original object, such as a portion of the human anatomy. Models are useful in teaching specific points. A model of the digestive tract is a valuable teaching aid in the review of anatomy and the description of the placement of the various stomas. Illustrations or photographs will convey the message, but a model gives a realistic approach to the teaching stubject.

Charts. The chart is a visual symbol for comparing, outlining, or arranging the subject matter in sequential interrelationships. The flow chart represents functional relationships in processes or events, designated by lines, rectangles, circles, or other graphic representations showing the directional flow.

Flip charts are often used by the instructor to emphasize specific points of discussion. The newsprint pad is a large pad of writing paper, usually placed on a stand, on which the instructor may illustrate (at the time of presentation or in advance) the main points of discussion. As each point is discussed, the sheet may be flipped over to new material.

Graphs. A graph is a type of chart but is usually listed as a separate teaching aid. The most commonly used graphs are the curve, line, bar, dot, diagram, and pictorial.

Graphs are most useful in representing statistics. They represent the successive changes in a variable quantity or quantities. They can become quite complicated, and care should be taken to gear them to the student level.

Audiovisual media. Materials immediately at hand, although audiovisual, such as the chalkboard, graphs, charts, exhibits, and the like, are not usually considered in the same realm of the more sophisticated areas of instructional materials such as television, radio, slides, filmstrips, or videotapes. These are usually referred to as audiovisual aids.

Audiovisual aids are designed for use in the presentation of information to the learner. These media should *support,* not *supplant,* the human element in group teaching. As a support they are often used to provide curriculum content to the individual student who desires or needs to review some portion of the materials covered.

There are many types of audiovisual materials that may be utilized by the ostomy instructor. Commercially produced motion pictures, filmstrips, and specially prepared television programs are available as teaching aids. Slides, transparencies, and recordings may be inexpensively yet professionally produced within the training department of the facility. The videotape recorder-player is a popular teaching adjunct. Although initially expensive, it offers a great many advantages, since a training program may be videotaped at the time it is presented and then repeated immediately through instant replay. It is also valuable to the instructor as a rehearsal aid or to the lecturer for a practice session. It may be privately set, operated, noted, and the tape then erased. The tapes may be erased and reused many times, or a filmed program may be filed for future class use.

New developments in the audiovisual media are occurring daily, and many manufacturers regularly publish lists and reviews of educational aids.

Videotaping hints for speakers.* Many persons are apprehensive when they are being videotaped for the first time. Some are even more reluctant to be videotaped a second time if the first taping revealed uncomplimentary mannerisms such as distracting facial expressions and gestures, redundancy in words or phrases, and a seeming lack of self-confidence. If certain basic points are remembered, videotaping can be made less confusing for both the speaker and the cameraperson, thereby resulting in better quality pictures and a more interesting program. Even novice speakers may improve their performances, feel more at ease before the camera, and become more proficient in preparing lectures and demonstrations that are to be videotaped.

1. *Colors*
   a. Skirts and blouses of medium to dark shades of blue, green, wine, and purple are the most appropriate. Pale colors, especially yellow and white, have a washed-out appearance and should be avoided.
   b. Medium to dark shades of brown, gray, blue, green, maroon or wine, and gold are good photographic colors for jackets. Bold patterns seem to fill the screen and are very distracting.
2. *Jewelry.* Many professional actors and actresses wear bold, glittering jewelry or costumes that create taping problems for the producer. This can be compensated for by the use of sophisticated filming equipment. However, the average hospital videotaping equipment cannot handle these problems without loss of quality in the finished product.
   a. Wide watchbands, costume jewelry with large stones, dangling earrings, and

*From the instructional materials prepared by Reba Grubb and Jane Mueller for the Tucson Medical Center Education Department.

eyeglass frames that reflect light are especially distracting to an audience intent on gaining insight into a complex problem.

   b. The speaker should stand in front of a mirror before videotaping and be sure that earrings are properly attached to the ears, a tie is straight, a nonglitter necklace is in alignment. Sometimes a loose earring or a crooked tie attracts more attention than a demonstration.

3. *Lecture content*
   a. Materials should be organized in advance. This includes the lecture and any visual aids that will be used to emphasize objectives.
   b. An outline should be prepared for the cameraperson. An indication where slides, charts, demonstrations, or other aids will be used should be made.
   c. Enough pretaping time should be allowed to "set the stage" for best results in both presentation and taping.
4. *Writing on the chalkboard or flip chart*
   a. Listing or columnar writing should follow a U shape rather than the standard listing procedure. For example, listing should start on the top left of the chalkboard and continue downward (no further than the audience and camera can read comfortably), move directly across from the last entry in the first column to begin the second column from the *bottom,* and continue listing *up*. The television camera moves more smoothly down, across, and up rather than focusing down one column and then making a quick shift to focus down again on the second column.
   b. When writing with chalk, press firmly and use bold figures or letters so the camera can pick up clear lines.
   c. The writer should stand slightly sideways and not in front of what is being written. The audience should be able to see the figures as they are made.
   d. The speaker should not move too quickly away from the written words to write in another place. There should be a pause long enough for the camera to focus on what was first written.
5. *Demonstrations*
   a. White objects such as parts of a skeleton or a plastic ostomy appliance should not be demonstrated against a white or light-colored background. The green chalkboard is better than the white visual screen.
   b. Cards, charts, graphs, and other visuals should be placed on an easel to stabilize the object for reading clarity.
6. *Rehearsing*. A dress rehearsal is the ideal method of preparation. This can be a rehearsal at home or before the videocamera if it is available for a practice session. During rehearsal, the full lecture, including use of visual aids, should be practiced until the speaker acquires self-confidence in handling the objects.
   a. Excessive moving around when talking should be avoided. It is difficult for the cameraperson to follow a moving object smoothly.
   b. When using a carousel projector, the speaker should avoid any actions that might interfere with the light beam.
   c. The overhead projector is designed to allow the speaker freedom to emphasize points by visually underlining them while facing the audience, thus eliminating the need for a speaker to look at the screen while talking.
7. *During taping*. To make a point with the video audience, the speaker should have good eye contact with the camera. The red light on the camera indicates

that the camera is operating. However, the speaker's contact with the live audience should not be sacrificed for the camera. With practice, the speaker will be able to manage eye contact with both audience and camera without loss to either.

8. *Question and answer session following the lecture.* Audience questions are difficult for the videotape to identify clearly. The speaker should repeat all questions posed before responding. Being unable to hear the questions is very frustrating to the video viewer, since the answer will make little sense without a question.
9. *Being natural in front of the camera.* This will be easier if the speaker will keep in mind that being selected to speak is an indication that the programmer acknowledges his qualifications to present the material.

Instructor. The choice of an instructor may prove to be the controlling factor in the success of a program. The ostomy nurse is a qualified professional and, with some training in instructional techniques, should be capable of conducting programs.

In addition to the ostomy nurse, resource persons should be selected from the various disciplines such as nursing, nutrition, social work, education, and the medical/surgical staff physicians. The teacher's attitudes and the knowledge and efforts exerted in teaching will influence the students. Each group is unique, and each person in the group is unique. The following qualifications may assist the committee in the selection of an instructor. The individual should:

1. Have a thorough knowledge of the area of ostomy education assigned.
2. Be creative in preparing and presenting demonstrations.
3. Be receptive to new ideas.
4. Have experience with group teaching and be able to stimulate participation.
5. Be familiar with the newest methods, techniques, and equipment and be able to locate resources and materials.
6. Be able to work well with the adult learner.
7. Be skillful in imparting information.
8. Be able to evaluate the sessions.
9. Be willing to help the individual student.
10. Be sensitive to attitudes of the class.

A course that is a part of the nursing school curriculum must be taught by an individual who can meet the basic accreditation qualifications if the course is offered for college credit. These qualifications are stated in the requirements for personnel in each institution and level.

The instructor's approach to the students and to the material involved will vary with the program. The orientation program will require only a cursory treatment of the subject, but the in-depth course, whether at the in-service or nursing school level, will demand knowledge of the material to be covered and of the equipment and source materials used. The student population of an in-service training class may be diverse in educational experience, knowledge, position, and skill; the instructor should be familiar with these variables and select the approaches in methodology that will best accomplish the course objectives.

Any instruction involving the learning of procedures and skills that the student will be expected to perform should allow the student an opportunity to develop his practical skill in class. Instruction in practical application of procedures and skills should include the following steps:

1. An explanation of the task and the procedures involved, offered in a step-by-step manner
2. Illustration of the task and the procedures involved (also performed step by step)
3. Student participation in the performance of the task with the instructor's assistance
4. Questions and answers and general discussion regarding specific problems encountered by the students
5. Student performance of the task without assistance

Efforts of students should be recognized as they participate in class and attempt to gain new skills. Achievement may be rewarded by some relative grading system or by the presentation of certificates.

A well-informed instructor who has a personal interest in the subject matter and an awareness of the scope of the program and the goals involved will gain the respect of the students and be able to effectively assist their learning processes.

Students. Any hospital personnel who are directly or indirectly involved in care of the ostomy patient will qualify as students for some level of ostomy training.

Nursing schools provide facilities of clinical practice, but the students are often assigned to hospitals in the community for experience in special fields such as ostomy. Personnel from other hospitals in the area are usually invited to attend ostomy programs, since this field is unique.

Scheduling. Some programs adapt readily to busy schedules, whereas others require more complex scheduling. Short absences from the unit may be tolerated. However, a day's absence will require a replacement.

The head nurses usually determine the scheduling of personnel for educational activities and plan in advance for staff coverage. Personnel should be released if at all possible at the time scheduled.

Programs should be scheduled to avoid overloading one week. Plans made well in advance will enable the staff to more effectively schedule personnel time off. Consideration should be given to appropriately accommodate the different shifts.

Checklists. Checklists of various responsibilities promote a more organized approach to planning. The lists will vary from the simple to the complex, from written notes on scrap paper to the formal printed plan, but whatever the form, planners will rely heavily on checklists. The following examples of checklists are all pertinent to programming.

Equipment, accessories, supplies

EQUIPMENT
- Tables
- Chairs
- Podium
- Chalkboards
- Easels
- Projectors
- Transparencies
- Videotapes
- Slides
- Tape recorders
- Models (for demonstration)
- Objects (beds, appliances, for demonstrations)

ACCESSORIES
- Place for hats and coats
- Adequate electric outlets
- Extension cords
- Room clock
- Microphones

SUPPLIES
- Masking tape
- Grease pencils
- Marking pens

SUPPLIES—cont'd
- Chalk
- Erasers
- Pointers
- Pads
- Pencils
- Evaluation forms
- Printed programs
- Newsprint pads
- Name tags
- Maps
- Material for distribution
- Attendance records
- Certificates
- Reimbursement slips
- Pitcher and glass
- Water for speaker
- Refreshment supplies
  - Coffee
  - Cups
  - Spoons
  - Cream
  - Sugar
  - Napkins

Checklist for session planning

1. Begin and end sessions on time.
2. Organize material in a logical manner.
3. Avoid long introductions.
4. Present one point at a time and complete it before introducing another.
5. Do not overload the sessions.
6. Fill in gaps with discussion.

Checklist for program coordinator

1. Consult with all department supervisors involved and discuss recommendations.
2. Contact speakers or instructors.
3. Reconfirm each commitment a week before the program and make arrangements for specific aids requested by the speaker.
4. Prepare handout material.
5. Immediately before the program review physical arrangements checklist.

6. Prepare a map (usually necessary for regional meetings), indicating location of conference area, restaurants, accommodations, tours.
7. Determine type of publicity and arrange for releases.
8. Send advance program to all participants.
9. Make sure all equipment is operable.
10. After meeting send appreciation notes to each guest speaker.
11. Evaluate and analyze the reaction to the program and send a copy to the administrator.

Physical arrangements. The planning committee will usually designate a physical arrangements chairman. The chairman is generally responsible for obtaining the necessary equipment and supplies for each program.

An atmosphere conducive to learning involves adequate facilities that are comfortable, generally accessible, and as free as possible from distracting surroundings. Learning is difficult when the classroom is overcrowded. Fire regulations, room temperature, ventilation, lighting, and restroom facilities are also essential considerations in planning for any size group.

Seating arrangements may vary, depending on the size of the group, type of program, and method of presentation. If written assignments are involved, tables and chairs or chairs with desk arms will be more comfortable.

The demonstration atmosphere is usually improved if students are seated in a semicircle, thereby allowing a clearer view of the demonstration.

Publicity. Advertisement of the program may be accomplished through the hospital's house organ, distribution of memoranda, or notices on the bulletin board. Community publicity may be given through newspapers, television, or radio. A comprehensive program may be announced over the public address system at the time of presentation.

Outlining the program. Ostomy education programs are tailored to fit specific purposes and priorities, identified by the evidence of needs. When these purposes have been established and the priorities set, the planning committee (or delegate) may begin outlining the program.

The outline may be altered many times before it is finalized. Basic outlines may serve many types of programs as long as they remain flexible and allow adaptation to new situations, new groups, and new ideas.

The following suggested outline is similar to the detail required by most advisory committees, administrative personnel, and accreditation boards.

1. Title
2. Course description
3. Objectives
4. Summary of content
5. Description of students
6. Credits offered
7. Time allotment (length of course, number of hours)
8. Methodology and training aids
9. Instructional materials

10. Facilities (arrangements)
11. Instructors
12. Outline of program (worksheet for each program)
13. Evaluation

The outline for the college course can be basically the same whatever the level at which it might be taught; however, the emphasis in the daily lesson plans, the field experience, detail, and so forth will vary. Colleges and universities across the country are not uniform in their course requirements, and instructional personnel develop independent lesson plans.

Program worksheet. A program worksheet is valuable in outlining each session or unit of the course. The layout of the worksheet is an individual preference. Most worksheets include the objectives of the session, method, and assignment. A more complete worksheet design will include all aspects of program planning, including evaluation.

Types of training programs. Following are basic plans for various types of training sessions.

ORIENTATION

The orientation program should be a broad coverage of the ostomy services that are available within the hospital.

OBJECTIVES

1. To acquaint new personnel with the facilities and services available to the ostomy patient
2. To identify opportunities for specialized training in the ostomy field

CONTENT

Introduction to the ostomy service should include information as to the location of the clinic (or office of the ostomy specialist if there is no clinic) and a general picture of the ostomy program in the hospital:

1. What is ostomy?
2. How prevalent is the need for ostomy care?
3. What personnel are involved in the patient's care?
4. What is ostomy's place in the overall institutional plan?

IN-SERVICE TRAINING—PROFESSIONAL

The professional in-service training course should be a presentation of current information relating to the ostomate population, ostomy needs, and caring for the hospitalized patient. Emphasis should be placed on procedures and skills in ostomy care and the practical application of those involved.

OBJECTIVES

1. To promote a better understanding of the ostomy patient
2. To increase familiarity with surgical procedures
3. To increase proficiency with ostomy collection appliances
4. To identify the ostomy patient's nutritional needs
5. To bring the results of research into clinical nursing practice

CONTENT
1. A brief review of the intestinal tract
2. Description of ostomy surgeries
3. Techniques of ostomy care
4. Attitudes and the nursing approach
5. Routine and emergency procedures
6. Advantages of modified diets
7. Ostomy terminology
8. Pathologic aspects of ostomy

IN-SERVICE TRAINING—NONPROFESSIONAL

The nonprofessional course will be less involved and require less time because some procedures and skills would not apply to this group. This course should present basics of ostomy service—understanding the patient and providing comforts and a pleasing atmosphere for him.

OBJECTIVES
1. To prepare the personnel to participate with greater understanding in ancillary care of the patient
2. To encourage personnel to recognize the patient's problems and develop a more sympathetic attitude
3. To develop an understanding of their role in care of the patient

CONTENT

Nursing service
1. General discussion of ostomy service
2. Basic ostomy anatomy
3. Demonstrations on how to move the patient
4. Demonstrations on how to bathe the patient
5. Discussion of attitudes and why patients respond emotionally as they do
6. Odor control
7. Ostomy terminology

Dietary service
1. Discussion of nutritional needs during illness
2. Emotions and their effect on the ability to eat
3. Basic anatomy of the gastrointestinal tract
4. Ostomy terminology

Housekeeping or environmental services
1. General discussion of ostomy service
2. Esthetic contribution to the well-being of the ostomy patient
3. Odor control

NURSING SCHOOLS, PRACTICAL NURSE TRAINING SCHOOLS, OSTOMY TRAINING SCHOOLS

This course is aimed toward the acquisition of special knowledge in procedures and nursing skills needed for the care of the ostomy patient. All areas of ostomy care should be explored, with emphasis on the nurse's or the ostomy therapist's role. This course attempts to create thinking for a positive future action in this field.

Clinical laboratory experience will be provided under the supervision and guidance of the instructor. The student will learn to formulate, implement, and evaluate nursing care plans for an assigned patient.

Case study will be an important adjunct to this course.

OBJECTIVES

1. To provide the student with an understanding of ostomy procedures and skills necessary to care for the ostomy patient
2. To familiarize the student with the fundamentals of ostomy, ostomy surgeries, recording of information, and utilization of available resources
3. To provide the student with an understanding of the ostomy patient and his particular physical and emotional problems
4. To enable the student to plan a diet, select and use appliances for the patient, and be alert to the problems of skin excoriation, fluid balance, and medications
5. To provide the student with the opportunity to examine existing methods of ostomy care
6. To provide the student with a basis for future research and innovation in the field

CONTENT

The course should include detailed study of the fundamentals of ostomy, care of the patient, recording of the information, and resources available in the field. Emphasis will be placed on the procedures and skills involved in ostomy care. The studies will include an introduction to ostomy services, anatomy (a brief review), ostomy surgeries, counseling, preoperative and postoperative care, care of the dying patient, skin care, selection and use of appliances, diet, medications, recording, community resources, and related services. An emphasis should be placed on new methods and equipment and the encouragement of reference reading. Emotional and physical rehabilitation will be an important consideration in this course.

WORKSHOPS OR CONFERENCES

The basic reason for either a conference or workshop is to explore a broad vital subject or problem more thoroughly than can be accomplished in meetings or occasional discussions.

It is a group learning process in which all types of methods of instruction may be utilized. The atmosphere is mentally stimulating, and participants learn by working and talking together, drawing on each other's experience and on reference materials. Capable leadership is vital to the workshop learning experience.

Several related subjects may be considered in a workshop, depending on the time allotment, but it is important that one subject be thoroughly discussed and completed before another subject is introduced. A review of all subjects should be given at the end of the course.

OBJECTIVES

1. To keep the ostomy nurse, stoma technician, and those who work with the ostomy patient well informed and up to date in the field

2. To disseminate information via the well-informed ostomy specialist to the institutions and agencies involved in the care of the ostomy patient throughout the world
3. To provide new ideas and information from which the ostomy patient can draw to help himself
4. To encourage professional personnel to participate more fully in the ostomy field

CONTENT

The content is based on continuing education in the care of the ostomy patient. The emphasis should be placed on new scientific discoveries, new ostomy surgeries or surgical methods, procedures and skills recently developed in the care of the patient, current dietary information, new medications and supplies, fluids and electrolyte balance, and skin care. Particular attention should be given to the constantly changing nature of the field of the ostomy specialist. New resources, attitudes, and ideas should be reviewed.

MEETINGS

Meetings, either community, regional, or national, will require careful, long-range planning. The planning committee will actively function throughout the planning process, meeting, and evaluation. Most national and regional meetings are governed by specific policies and procedures, with certain areas of planning delegated to the local groups. Experts on the regional and national levels are usually available for consultation.

All areas of the planning process must be considered.

OBJECTIVES

1. To bring together persons with a common interest, to review, plan, and discuss developments concerning ostomy
2. To review the results of research in order to effectively utilize all new developments that are appearing
3. To develop an understanding of the scope of ostomy surgeries, current statistical data, and future plans

OPPORTUNE TEACHING

The opportunity for learning activities occurs often during the daily work routine on the unit. These person-to-person instructions contribute to higher standards of patient care since they are taught at the time a need is evidenced. The effective ostomy specialist should take advantage of the opportune situation as it occurs. Practical knowledge is often gained during coffee breaks, committee meetings, or chance encounters in the corridors, library, or lounge.

PUBLIC SCHOOL HEALTH CAREERS EDUCATION

The health careers projects are designed to give selected high school students who have completed their junior year an opportunity to explore several areas in the health field. The project allows them to become familiar with hospital routine by actual participation in various departments throughout the hosptial. If sufficiently motivated, the students may continue in an organized health careers program during their senior year.

CONTINUING EDUCATION

Participation in a continuing education program is on a voluntary basis. Personnel who desire additional learning are motivated to add to their abilities and to elevate their knowledge of developments in the health field. The in-service or nursing school level courses should be offered on a continuing basis, with emphasis on new developments in research, equipment, and appliances. Nursing personnel should be encouraged to attend workshops and regional and national meetings. A reimbursement of cost should be absorbed by the hospital is possible.

Evaluation. Evaluation is a process through which specific criteria are utilized to measure formally and/or informally the degree to which stated objectives have been reached. In ostomy education the process is important in assessing the effectiveness of programs, meetings, course content, instructor or speaker performance, student performance in a particular context, on-the-job skills, and many other related activities. It should be considered an important element in the planning process, since the design for improving future programs and the indication of additional needs may be derived from the results of an evaluation analysis.

To be considered valid, evaluation criteria must assess whether the original objectives have been met, regardless of the subject being evaluated. For example, one objective of an orientation program is to acquaint new personnel with the facilities and services available to the ostomy patient. If the orientation program is to be evaluated, a portion of the criteria must assess whether this objective has been achieved. Some questions that are usually valid considerations in establishing evaluation criteria are noted below in several subject areas.

Evaluation of a speaker

1. Did the presentation indicate that the speaker was adequately prepared?
2. Was the speech geared to the student level?
3. What teaching methods and training aids were used?
4. Was the speaker effective? Dynamic? Weak?
5. Did the person hold the interest of the group?
6. Was the subject matter clearly understood by the students?
7. Did the speaker adequately cover the subject assigned?
8. Did the individual involve the group? If so, how?
9. Would you ask this speaker for a return engagement?

Evaluation of materials

All teaching materials should be reviewed before they are presented and evaluated after they are utilized.

1. Did the material contribute meaningful content to the topic?
2. Was it appropriate for the student level?
3. Did the material merit the time and expense involved?
4. Did it stimulate interest?

Evaluation of the program

An evaluation of any educational project is an important method of measuring its effectiveness.

1. Did it achieve its objectives?
2. Did it offer worthwhile information?
3. Did it stimulate interest in ostomy?
4. Did it change attitudes toward stoma stigmas?
5. Did it help to develop higher standards of patient care?
6. Did it interpret the hospital's ostomy program?
7. How effective were the speakers? Did they convey the intended message?
8. Was there ample opportunity for audience participation?
9. Was there a cooperative spirit?

Student's evaluation of the course

1. What did you like best about this program?
2. What did you dislike about the program?
3. What speaker was the most effective? Why?
4. Did the material presented offer new thoughts or ideas for better job performance?
5. Was the course applicable to your particular interests?
6. What would have made the course more effective?
7. On the whole, how do you rate this program? Poor? Mediocre? Good? Excellent?

Evaluation of workshop or conference

1. If there were speakers, which one impressed you the most? Why? Which one impressed you the least? Why?
2. Did the program's design meet your particular need or interest?
3. What ideas or suggestions did you gain from the meeting that will be useful to you and other personnel in your work performance?
4. Were the time and monetary investments worthwhile?

CHAPTER 3

Anatomic and physiologic overview

A working knowledge of the structure and functions of body systems is important to the nurse who must assess and teach the ostomy patient. Since this material usually is included in general nursing education, it is not new to the nurse practitioner. It is the purpose of this chapter to provide a brief overview of the structure and functions of some of the body systems, offering the ostomy nurse an opportunity for review.

ALIMENTARY CANAL

Nourishment is taken into the body through the mouth and carried through the body by means of the alimentary canal, a tube lined with mucous membrane and comprising the entire digestive system. During digestion, food must be reduced to a fluid state. This process begins in the mouth, where the food is ground with the teeth and then pushed backward by the tongue into the pharynx, where the act of swallowing is initiated.

The *pharynx,* commonly called the throat, is a muscular bag about 4 inches in length. It is located behind the nasal cavity and the mouth and extends from the base of the skull to the esophagus. Food is squeezed through a pharyngeal opening into the esophagus.

The *esophagus* is a muscular tube approximately 9 inches long that connects the pharynx with the stomach. The rings of this muscular tube contract and force food into the stomach through an opening called the cardiac sphincter. This contraction within the body is achieved by peristaltic waves, which are controlled by vagal reflexes.

The *stomach* is a conical enlargement of the alimentary canal located between the esophagus and the small intestine. It is about 12 inches in length and 5 inches in diameter. It is composed of a layer of muscle covered with peritoneum and lined with mucous membrane. The stomach membrane contains gastric glands that daily secrete almost 3 quarts of a special digestive fluid called gastric juice. Gastric juice contains hydrochloric acid and two ferments: rennin, a coagulant, and pepsin, which softens the albumin of food. Gastric juice slowly eats its way into the food mass, dissolving the cells that compose the food. Through peristalsis, food flows in a steady stream from the esophagus to the stomach, where it makes a circuit of the stomach in approximately 3 minutes and thoroughly mixes with gastric juice. Living germs of fermentation and disease are sometimes swallowed. The acid in the gastric juice, if in full amount, prevents food from spoiling and acts as a disinfectant.

The result of stomach digestion is a thin, milky fluid called chyme, to which peptone gives a bitter taste. The stomach is not absolutely necessary for digestion, but because of its capacity, it serves as a storehouse for food and eliminates the need for eating every few minutes.

The *pylorus,* the distal aperture of the stomach, opens and closes at intervals to permit a little chyme to escape into the intestine, where the main work of digestion is performed. The pyloric valve prevents the return of food to the stomach.

From 2 to 5 hours are required to completely empty the stomach, depending on the amount of food and the ease with which it is broken up. When the stomach is empty, there is a feeling of hunger, although the intestines may contain enough digested food to supply the body for hours.

The part of the alimentary canal below the stomach is a tube of varying size, with each portion having a different name. The *small intestine,* which adjoins the stomach, is 1 inch in diameter and approximately 20 feet long. It opens into the *large intestine,* which is about 2 inches in diameter and 5 feet long.

Most of the nutrition absorption occurs in the small intestine during a period 8 to 12 hours after eating. The small intestine is very movable and is coiled in the abdomen. It is attached to the spinal column by a fold of mesentery. In front of the intestines is a thin apron called omentum, which contains fat and acts as a cushion and a protection.

The small intestine has three divisions. There are no evident marks of separation as they merge imperceptibly into each other; however, internal characteristics serve to distinguish the divisions. Beginning at the stomach, approximately the first 10-inch section of the small intestine is called the *duodenum.* The next 8-foot section is the *jejunum,* and the remaining 11-foot section is the *ileum.*

Internally, the small intestine contains folds called valvulae conniventes. These prevent food from passing through the intestine too quickly and present a greater surface for the absorption of the digested food. On the surface of each fold are fingerlike projections called villi. Between the bases of the villi are minute tubes extending into the mucous membrane. Each tube secretes a small amount of intestinal juice containing ferments that change starch to glucose and albumin to peptone, but this digestive action is slight.

The small intestine opens into the side of the large intestine from the ileum to the cecum by means of the ileocecal valve, which permits matter to pass into the large intestine and prevents its backward movement.

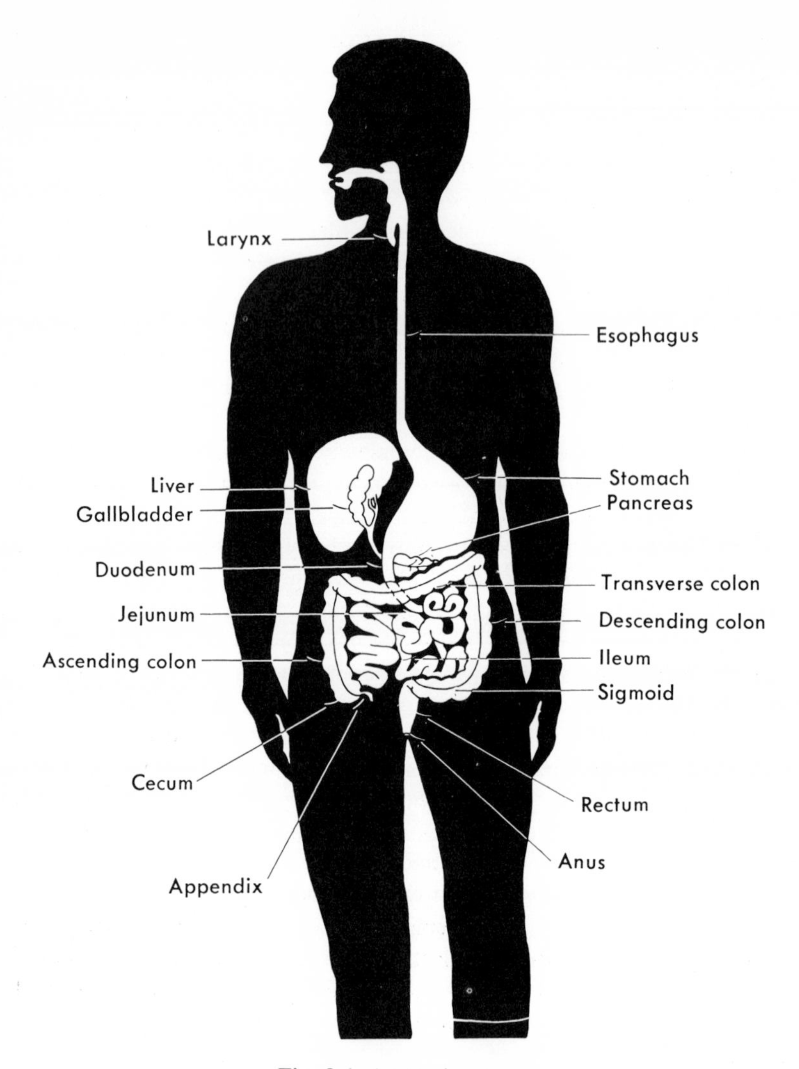

Fig. 3-1. Anatomic areas.

The large intestine is known as the *colon*. It is not an even tube; rather it looks as though strings were tied about it every few inches. It begins with the *cecum,* a blind pouch projecting downward below the ileocecal junction. A small tube, variable in length (2 to 6 inches), is attached to the cecum below the ileocecal opening; this is called the vermiform appendix. The *ascending colon* extends upward from the ileocecal junction to the right hepatic flexure. The *transverse colon* extends in a loop from the hepatic flexure to the splenic flexure. The *descending colon* extends from the splenic flexure to the

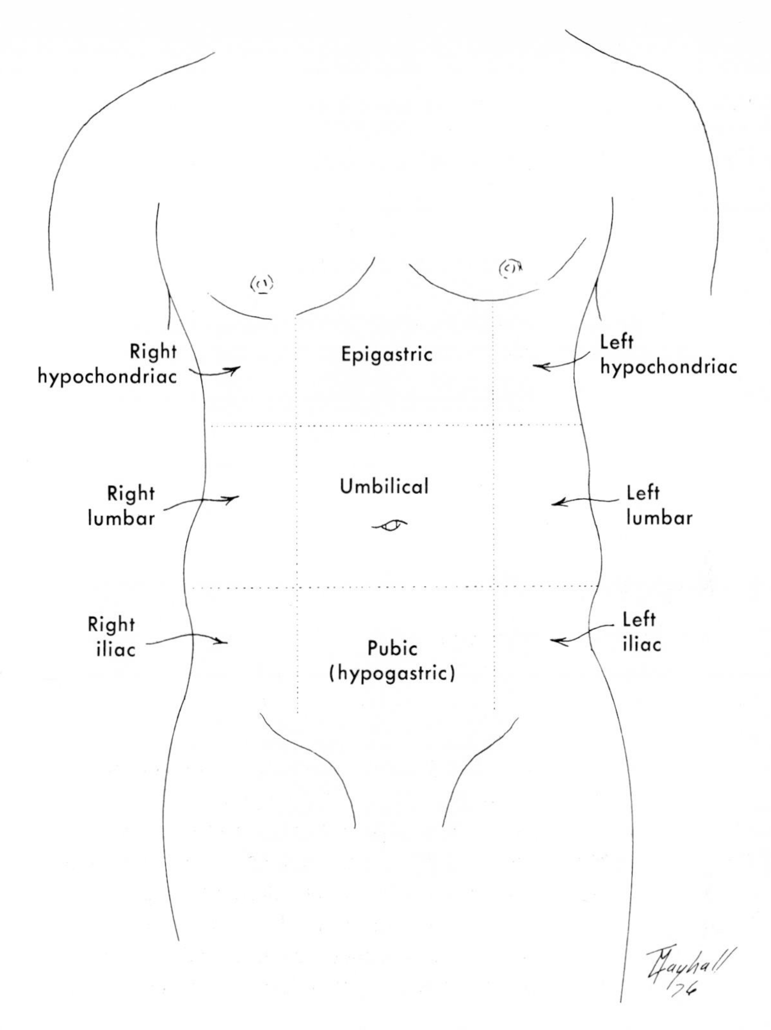

Fig. 3-2. The nine regions of the abdomen. (Courtesy Education Department, Tucson Medical Center.)

S-shaped *sigmoid colon,* which leads into the *rectum,* the last and nearly straight portion of the large intestine. The anus leads to the exterior of the body and is kept closed, except during defecation, by contraction of the involuntary circular muscle known as the external sphincter. The digestive process in the large intestine takes approximately 36 hours.

Bands called taeniae coli form the ligaments of the colon as they run from the cecum to the rectum, and they present a striking contrast to the smooth cylindrical contour of the wall of the intestine.

ACCESSORY ORGANS TO THE DIGESTIVE PROCESS

The accessory organs—liver, pancreas, and gallbladder—empty juices into the duodenum through the ampulla of Vater.

The *pancreas* is a gland about 1 inch in diameter and 6 to 8 inches long that lies behind the stomach. It secretes a thin watery liquid called pancreatic juice, which pours into the duodenum at the rate of 1½ pints a day. Pancreatic juice is made up of three ferments that perform the main part of digestion. As the chyme enters the intestines, it contains albumin, some already digested but much of it only softened and broken up. These ferments act on the chyme: trypsin acts on the digested albumin, changing it to peptone; amylopsin changes the starch to glucose; and steapsin acts as a lubricating and cleansing agent.

The *liver* lies under the lowest ribs on the right side of the body. It secretes bile, which is collected by biliary ducts and carried to the duodenum during digestion. On the underside of the liver is a pear-shaped organ about 4 inches long and 1 inch wide, the *gallbladder*. This organ stores bile when the intestine does not need it.

URINARY SYSTEM

The urinary system, often compared to a filtering plant, is a mechanism by which the body's soluble waste is converted into urine and eliminated. This system consists of two kidneys, two ureters, the urinary bladder, and the urethra.

The *kidneys* are paired tubular glands approximately 4 inches long, 2 inches wide, and 1 inch thick. These very complex organs are reddish brown in color, shaped like lima beans, and situated in the posterior part of the lumbar region of the abdomen, one on either side of the spinal column. Blood enters the kidney by means of the renal arteries and is filtered through numerous fine tubes made up of epithelial cells. The purified blood returns to the body's circulation system and the waste products are eventually drained into the kidney pelvis, or sac, where muscle contraction forces the urine down the ureters.

The *ureters* are two mucous membrane-lined muscular tubes approximately 12 to 18 inches long. They serve as a channel for the urine to flow from the kidneys into the urinary bladder.

The *urinary bladder* is a large hollow muscular organ lined with mucous membrane and amply supplied with blood, lymph vessels, and nerves. In the female it is situated in front of the anterior wall of the vagina and neck of the uterus, and in the male it is in front of the rectum. The urinary bladder serves as a reservoir for the urine until it is expelled from the body through the urethra.

The *urethra* is a narrow muscular tube lined with mucous membrane. It connects the urinary bladder to the body's exterior orifice, the urinary meatus, and has the ability of considerable dilation. The male urethra measures 8 or 9 inches in length while the female urethra's approximate length is only 1½ inches.

The body excretes an average of 1½ quarts of urine daily, through the act of micturition.

LARYNX

The larynx is a triangular box approximately ¾ inch across that connects the trachea and pharynx. It is composed of nine bands of fibrocartilages. Two thin fibrous bands are stretched across the upper end of the larynx. Air passing between these bands produces the voice.

INTEGUMENTARY SYSTEM

The skin is the major organ of the integumentary system. Included in the system are oil glands, sweat glands and ducts, nails, and hairs of the body. Human skin undergoes constant change and renewal. Skin thickness varies as does skin appearance, which varies according to age and race.

The skin functions as a mechanical barrier to microorganisms, as a sense organ, as an important factor in heat regulation, as an excretory organ, as an absorbing organ, and as a respiratory organ.

CIRCULATORY SYSTEM

The circulatory system is a complex irrigation system concerned with the transportation of fluid from one part of the body to another. The system consists of two divisions: the blood or vascular system, consisting of the heart, arteries, capillaries, and veins; and the lymphatic system, including the lacteals and ducts and lymphatic nodes and glands.

The arteries are the vessels that carry the blood away from the heart. They decrease progressively in size as they divide. The capillaries convey the blood from the arteries to the veins. They usually form networks in the tissues. The veins are the vessels that carry blood to the heart. The walls of the veins are thinner than those of the corresponding arteries.

The blood serves several purposes in the body:

1. It carries material, including water, oxygen, and certain glandular secretions to the tissues.
2. It takes away from the tissues the waste products to be eliminated by the kidneys, lungs, and skin.
3. It distributes and equalizes heat produced in the tissues by oxidation.
4. It contains certain constituents that aid in protecting the body from bacteria and other foreign substances.

REPRODUCTIVE ORGANS

The primary functions of the reproductive organs in both the male and female are identical—continuation of human life through procreation and achievement of sexual gratification. The male internal organs include two testes, two epididymides, two seminal ducts and vesicles, two ejaculatory ducts, two spermatic cords, the urethra, the prostate, and other glands. External reproductive organs are the glans penis and scrotum.

The female internal reproductive organs include the uterus (womb), two fallopian tubes, two ovaries, and the vagina. External genitals, referred to as the vulva, are the mons pubis, labia majora and minora, clitoris, vestibule, hymen, and several glands.

CENTRAL NERVOUS SYSTEM

The central nervous system is the communication system of the body. It is the nerve center of man and therefore responsible for all that man is and all that he does. The major organs of the central nervous system are the brain and the spinal cord. The many nerve branches leading from the cord are essential to its function. Cerebrospinal fluid and membranes, called meninges, surround the brain and cord and add protection by cushioning them. The basis of the nervous system, as with other systems, is the cell or neuron, which carries out its function of communication.

Major functions of the central nervous system are control of consciousness, control of mental processes, regulation of body movements and functions, and transmission and reception of nerve impulses to all areas of the body.

This system is subdivided into the sympathetic and parasympathetic nerves. The voluntary nervous system responds to the conscious will. The autonomic or involuntary nervous system works automatically as it conducts impulses to the heart muscle, smooth muscles of the blood vessels, digestive organs, and other organs and glands with nervous impulses.

The sympathetic and parasympathetic nerves influence the muscular activity of the gastrointestinal organs. The sympathetic reaches through the splanchnic nerve and the parasympathetic, which are derived from the medulla oblongata in the brain, pass through the vagus nerve, and act on the muscles of the stomach, small intestine, and proximal half of the large intestine. Other parasympathetic nerves, branching from the sacral portion, supply the lower half of the large intestine and rectum.

CHAPTER 4

From symptoms to surgery

SYMPTOMS

The process of eating is designed to furnish the body with adequate nourishment. Simple foods eaten in desirable amounts and at regular intervals suited to the individual body will allow the digestive mechanism to function properly.

Eating habits that include fast ingestion and excessive amounts disturb the stomach. Symptoms of an abused stomach are headache, rapid heartbeat, nausea, diarrhea, fever, pain, gas, or indigestion. Gases distend the stomach, and the diaphragm exerts pressure on the heart, sometimes confusing a digestive upset with cardiovascular problems. If the cause of these symptoms is not removed, actual stomach distress can result, causing serious diseases for which surgery may be the only answer.

Fatigue without an obvious cause is a danger signal. A sudden or extreme change in body weight, bowel habits, skin, or personality needs investigating. Hemorrhaging from a body opening, lumps or growths in any part of the body, loss of appetite, and swelling in the abdomen are all symptoms that should be explored.

The family physician may refer a patient with complicated symptoms to either the internist or the gastroenterologist, a specialist in diseases that affect the digestive tract and related systems.

A thorough background history of the patient is important to successful diagnosis. It helps to identify causes such as hereditary diseases, the patient's habits over a long period of time, accidents, or early illnesses that might have contributed to the present condition.

After completing the history and examining the patient, the specialist will decide and schedule diagnostic tests or procedures for the patient.

DIAGNOSTIC TESTS OR PROCEDURES

Illness must be diagnosed and the cause of disease determined before any operative procedure can be decided. The frustration of treating only what they could see led early physicians to experiment with various methods of diagnosing disease. Such experimentation resulted in the development of procedures for diagnosing the need for ostomy surgery and in the design of instruments or scopes that can be inserted in various openings of the body for internal viewing.

Common diagnostic tests and examinations, used to help establish a diagnosis for the ostomy patient, may be performed in the physician's office or a diagnostic center; however, the patient may be hospitalized for diagnosis of severe symptoms.

Prior explanation to the patient of the procedures to be performed and the necessary preparation is essential to gaining his understanding and cooperation. Diagnosticians usually give the patient a printed explanation of the procedure and answer questions the patient may have.*

Diagnosing by means of radiology

Barium enema. Lesions, diverticuli, polyps, and fistulas are easily visualized by using barium studies. Barium is a white, chalklike liquid that is inserted through a rectal tube. An important factor in successful pictures is whether the bowel has been throughly cleansed prior to the examination. Fluoroscopy with barium demonstrates peristaltic abnormalities.

Intravenous pyelogram. The intravenous pyelogram (IVP) visualizes the bladder and kidney through the aid of a dye injected into the vein. Radiographs of the urinary tract will detect kidney stones, kinked ureters, or malfunctioning kidneys.

Gastrointestinal series. In this procedure barium is swallowed to aid in the detection of ulceration or tumor in the stomach and duodenum. The barium is seen by x-ray photography as it travels, outlining the esophagus, stomach wall, and duodenum. Physicians often order laxatives to eliminate barium residue from the intestines after the test is completed.

Radiographic examinations. An ostomy patient frequently returns to the hospital or to an outpatient clinic for x-ray examinations that may be used in the diagnosis of a complication or an evaluation of a loop colostomy for possible closure. Ileostomy patients rarely require barium enemas.

The colon is usually evaluated by the instillation of barium through the stoma. This situation presents special problems, since the stoma, unlike the anus, has no sphincter; therefore barium solutions tend to leak onto the abdominal wall.

When removal of the rectum is deferred, or if the rectum is retained as a defunctional stump, the physician may desire to examine this portion of the colon. In this study the barium is instilled through the rectum.

Preparation of the colon is important for clear films. It must be clean and free of bismuth preparations. Patients who use such preparations should be instructed to discontinue them at least 3 days prior to the examination.

To accomplish a successful barium enema on the ostomy patient with

---

*The test protocols are descriptive only and are not intended to be complete.

minimal discomfort and stress, an irrigator cone may be used to instill the barium solution and prevent leakage.

The Greer No. 6090 hospital pack irrigation appliance is a good example of an irrigator set with a cone. It has a self-adhering sleeve, an irrigating bag with tubing and cone attached, and spring clamps for regulation of the flow.

Procedure for inpatient

1. Remove the patient's appliance.
2. Cleanse and dry the skin circumostomy.
3. Remove the adhesive protective paper.
4. Hold the sleeve with the short end toward the patient's head. Center the stoma in the aperture and adhere the sleeve to the patient. Avoid wrinkles in the adhesive.
5. Approximate the bottom of the sleeve to the top, fold together, and

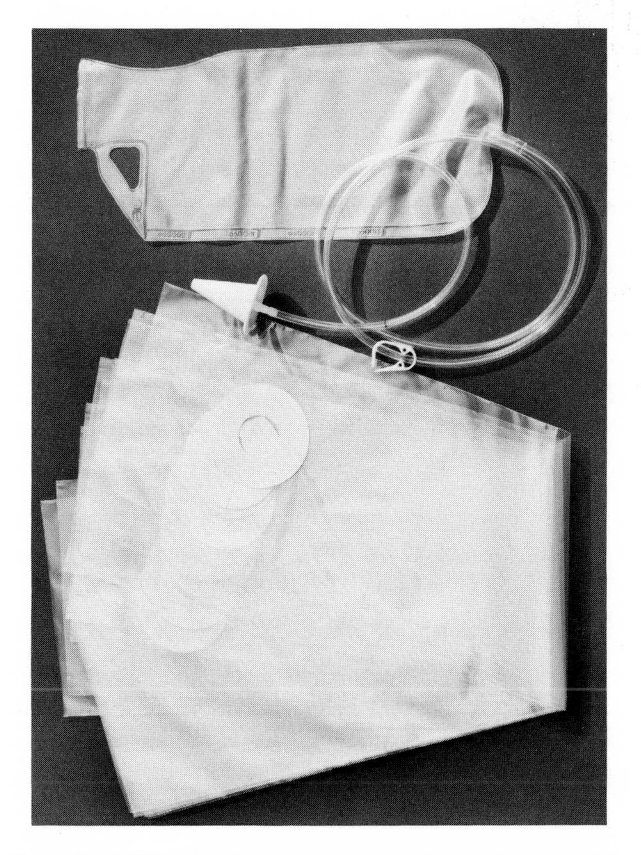

Fig. 4-1. Greer No. 6090 hospital pack irrigation appliance. (Courtesy John F. Greer Co.)

hold with a spring clamp. Send the irrigator along with the patient to the x-ray department.
6. In the x-ray department, fill the irrigator with barium solution. Clamp the tubing and hang the irrigator on a standard.
7. Clear the air from the tubing by opening the clamp and allowing a small amount of barium to run through the tubing.
8. Lubricate the cone.
9. Introduce the cone from the top of the sleeve and then *gently* insert it into the stoma. Some stomas readily admit the cone, but when there is a problem with stenosis, the cone must not be forced. The cone will block the backflow of the barium with partial insertion.
10. When the patient is able to assist, instruct him to hold the cone in place. If necessary, the cone may be secured with tape. Securing the cone is important, since the patient's body will be moved from side to side during the examination.
11. When the x-ray films are completed, remove the cone.
12. Bring the bottom of the sleeve to the top and clamp the two edges together. Leave the sleeve in place.
13. Return the irrigator and cone with the inpatient to his room.
14. As soon as the patient has rested, any remaining barium should be removed to prevent any chance of opaque concretion. The regular colostomy irrigation procedure is used.

Procedure for outpatient. The outpatient may be instructed to replace the regular appliance with the irrigator sleeve before coming to the clinic for a barium study.

At the conclusion of the examination, the outpatient may wish to irrigate before leaving the clinic and replace the irrigator sleeve with his own pouch. A room should be provided for this procedure.

Endoscopy*

Endoscopes are visual instruments that are used to diagnose and treat diseases within the body cavities. They may be introduced through natural body openings or through artificially constructed openings.

A special camera may be attached to these instruments to photograph the internal organs.

Routine preparations include nothing by mouth after midnight. Once in the examining room, the patient will be medicated as necessary and examined. If other procedures are necessary, the physician will fully explain them to the patient and administer the proper medications in order to continue further examinations. Any questionable sites are biopsied.

---

*The majority of the tests and procedures are from *Gastroenterology: Laboratory Manual* by John McGregor, M.D., gastroenterologist, Tucson Medical Center.

Peritoneoscopy and laparoscopy

Peritoneoscopy and laparoscopy are examinations of the interior of the abdomen. This visualization of the viscera can aid in establishing diagnosis and the planning of a surgical procedure.

Medications are administered according to the individual requirements. The procedure is performed in the operating room, where the visualizing instrument is inserted through a small incision.

Rectal examinations

Rectal examinations include digital examination, anoscopy, proctoscopy, and sigmoidoscopy. These are performed for symptoms of bleeding or any change in bowel habits. All four procedures are similar except in the area of examination: the digital and anoscopy examinations are used for the anal region, the proctoscopy reaches further into the rectum, and the sigmoidoscopy extends the examination to the sigmoid colon.

Colonoscopy

Colonoscopy is a diagnostic procedure used frequently in large bowel obstruction and utilized in the removal of colon-pedunculated polyps and biopsies. With the development of the pliable and more easily controlled colonoscope, it is now possible to reach the full length of the large intestine in most patients. Scopes are illuminated by a cold light source and have a fiberoptic magnifying lens system that permits examination of the inside of the colon in great detail. Also, by attaching a 35 mm camera to the instrument, color photographs may be obtained. The tip of the instrument is equipped with an opening through which flexible biopsy forceps or a cautery snare for polyp removal may be introduced. There is also a passage for the introduction of air to inflate the bowel as well as an irrigation tube.

Before the insertion of the colonoscope, the colon must be cleaned and free of residue. This is accomplished according to the physician's preference. Elemental chemically defined diets, cathartics, and/or cleansing enemas may be used. *A clean colon is an important factor in obtaining an accurate examination.*

Following is an example of a procedure for the removal of polyps: The patient is placed on a clear liquid diet for 2 days and given laxatives and tap water enemas the evening before the procedure. Prior to the examination the patient is usually given a sedative to relieve apprehension and other medication to relax the colon. Examination is begun with the patient lying on his back with his knees bent. The scope is introduced through the rectum and guided into the colon. When the polyp is located, a wire snare is fed through the scope and looped around the stalk of the polyp. The wire is tightened, electrical current is applied for cauterization, and the polyp is separated from the colonic mucosa. As the scope is withdrawn, suction is applied and the polyp is drawn out. All parts of the colon are accessible, and during one procedure numerous polyps can be removed. Rarely do complications occur. The lack of discomfort to the patient is an obvious advantage.

Choledochoscopy

Choledochoscopy is the visualization and examination of the biliary tree through an incision in the common bile duct by means of a choledochoscope. Its principal use is in postcholedochotomy examination of the common and hepatic bile ducts. Bile, which is opaque, presents a visualization problem and must be diluted. The choledochoscope consists of two parts: the fiberoptic instrument for visualization and a semiflexible irrigation tube or cannula for the insertion of fluid to dilute the bile. Biopsy forceps or a cytology brush may be passed through the irrigation fluid channel.

Gastrointestinal tests

Esophageal hydrochloric acid perfusion test. This test assists in the differential diagnosis of chest pain. A positive test tends to confirm the diagnosis of esophagitis.

The patient should be instructed to have nothing by mouth after mignight on the day of the test. No anticholinergic medication, antacid medication, narcotics, or barbiturates should be taken for 12 hours prior to the test. No smoking should be allowed the morning of the test.

A nasogastric tube is passed into the upper esophagus. Normal saline solution, 0.1 N hydrochloric acid, or sodium bicarbonate is successively dripped into the patient's esophagus and the patient's response noted. The test will require approximately 1 hour.

Basal gastric secretory level (basal gastric acid output). This test determines the level of gastric secretory activity in the absence of known secretory stimuli, assists in the differentiation of the Zollinger-Ellison syndrome, and assists in the detection of achlorhydria.

The patient is instructed as for motility studies. A nasogastric tube is passed in such a fashion that the tip lies at or near the pylorus. If gastric surgery has been done or if there is any deformity of the stomach, the position of the tube is confirmed by fluoroscopy. The volumes of each specimen are recorded and reported. The test takes approximately 1½ hours.

Histalog stimulation study. The purpose of this study is to determine the presence or absence of achlorhydria, to quantitatively determine the secretory capacity of the stomach under a near-maximum stimulus, and to provide guidance for the type of proposed gastric surgery.

The patient should be instructed to take nothing by mouth for 12 hours prior to the test. Anticholinergic medication, narcotics, antacids, and smoking are proscribed for the same period of time. A nasogastric tube is placed in the stomach as for a basal gastric secretory test. The basal acid output is determined over a 30- to 60-minute period of time. The patient is then given betazole (Histalog), histamine, or pentagastrin in a dose that varies according to true body weight. The acid output under these test conditions is determined. The test will require approximately 2 hours.

Insulin stimulation study (Hollander test). This is a test to quantitatively assess the physiologic competency of vagus nerves and the completeness of surgical vagotomy.

The patient is instructed as for motility studies. A radiopaque nasogastric tube is placed in the stomach, usually under x-ray guidance. Two 15-minute aliquots of gastric aspirate are collected for basal acid output (BAO). A fasting blood sugar measurement is obtained. Regular insulin is given intravenously. Four consecutive 30-minute aliquots of gastric aspirate are collected over the next 120 minutes and tested for hydrogen ion concentration. Blood sugar measurements are obtained 45 and 120 minutes after giving insulin to ensure that blood sugar level drops below 45 mg/100 ml during the test period. Acid output is determined under these test conditions. The test requires approximately 3 hours.

Biliary drainage study (Lyon's drainage). Study of biliary tract drainage will often be of material assistance in the diagnosis of gallbladder or biliary tract diseases.

The patient is instructed as for motility studies. A Rehfuss tube is passed under fluoroscopic control so that its tip lies at a point just below the ampulla of Vater. The duodenal contents are siphoned off and retained. Magnesium sulfate solution is administered through the tube. ''A'' bile is collected by siphonage and suction and then ''B'' bile is collected. The specimens are microscopically examined, the volume of secretion is recorded, and the pH of the solutions is obtained. Cultures of the solutions may be done. Duration of the test is 1 to 1½ hours.

Malabsorption studies

Microscopic examination of stool for fat. This study provides a rapid qualitative test for detecting the presence of excess neutral fat in feces. A freshly defecated sample of feces is brought to the laboratory. A small aliquot of this sample is spread on a glass slide and stained with Sudan III or Sudan IV. The slide is then examined under the low-power objective of the microscope for red-stained globules of fat. If no fat is seen, glacial acetic acid is added to the slide and the slide is heated. The slide is then reexamined for stained neutral fat.

Quantitative determination of fecal fat content. This study provides a quantitative determination of neutral fat contained in a 72-hour fecal sample. Since fat is the most difficult substance to digest and absorb, excessive elimination of neutral fat is often the first sign of pancreatic or intestinal malfunction.

The patient should be started on a diet that contains between 70 to 100 gm of fat per day. Cooperation of the Dietary Department is important in monitoring the fat intake. Diet should be started 3 days prior to collection of feces.

The patient should not be taking any pancreatic enzyme, alcohol, bile salt preparation, or laxative medication.

While on the prescribed diet, all of the patient's feces are collected over a 72-hour period. The feces are then quantitatively assayed for total neutral fat content.

d-Xylose tolerance test. d-Xylose is an artificial sugar that is presumed to be absorbed in a fashion similar to glucose. Since it cannot be metabolized by the human organism, it can be used as an excellent quantitative measurement of carbohydrate absorption.

The patient is maintained in a fasting state for 12 hours prior to the test. A fasting, pretest blood sample is drawn for d-xylose level. A standard amount of d-xylose dissolved in water is given to the patient to drink, and subsequent blood levels of d-xylose are determined. Duration of the test is 2 hours.

Cytology

Cytologic examinations may be made during endoscopy procedures with a special brush and technique and then sent to the pathologist.

Pathology

Biopsies, smears, and specimens are sent to the pathologist, who prepares them for microscopic evaluation and notifies the physician of the results.

DISEASES OR CONDITIONS PREDISPOSING TO OSTOMY SURGERY

Certain symptoms bring the patient to the attention of the diagnostician. Following are examples of diseases associated with disorders that may require ostomy surgery:

Cancer of the larynx is a slowly growing tumor that tends to remain local for a very long time. Vocal cords may be easily examined and the tumor diagnosed and treated by radiation or surgery.

Polyposis of the colon is the presence of multiple polyps throughout the large bowel that sometimes develop into cancer. Polyposis is thought to be familial.

Crohn's disease, or transmural enterocolitis, is a nonspecific inflammatory bowel disease. It is very complex. The entire colon or only parts of it may be involved. The disease process may extend in continuity or skip areas. The term "transmural" describes one of the characteristics of the disease, since in many places it affects all layers of the bowel wall.

Hawk* has named some of the distinctive differences between ulcerative colitis and Crohn's disease (Table 1).

---

*Hawk, William A.: Primary inflammatory bowel disease, facts and fancy, Ostomy Quart. **11:**3-4, Fall, 1974.

Table 1. Distinctive differences between ulcerative colitis and Crohn's disease

Symptom	Ulcerative colitis	Crohn's disease
1. Ulcerations	Superficial	Deep and undermining
2. Fistulas and strictures	Unobserved	Relatively common
3. Granulomas	Never	Indication
4. Involvement of small intestine	Seldom more than 10 cm	Extensive
5. Cancer	Incidence reported in patients with long-standing involvement	Very casual association

Ulcerative colitis is usually curable by surgical removal of the colon and rectum. Recurrences of Crohn's disease may require further surgical intervention.

Cancer of the colon is a neoplasm or cellular tumor usually associated with a group of tumors. Early detection of the growth and its immediate removal offers a fairly good chance for cure.

Ulcerative colitis (irritable colon) is an acute or chronic inflammatory condition of the colon subject to remissions (abatement of symptoms) and exacerbations (increase in severity of symptoms). It is usually accompanied by diarrhea, nausea, vomiting, abdominal pain, fever, bleeding, and weight loss. The patient loses fluids and blood with the fecal discharge. Neither the cause nor the cure has yet been established.

Diverticulosis is a weakness of the muscle layers of the bowel wall causing an outpouching formation of small sacs, which become filled with feces, thereby setting up irritation and sometimes resulting in abscesses leading to fistula formations.

Ileitis is an inflammatory disease of the small intestine at the point where it joins the large intestine (ileocecal valve), with ulcerations present along the mucosa. The ulcerations may perforate and form fistulas, causing the formation of scar tissue as the fistula heals. This scar tissue may cause stricture and result in intestinal obstruction.

A *fistula* is an abnormal opening connecting either two hollow organs within the body or a hollow organ within the body to the outside.

Abdominal trauma may result from injuries caused by knives, bullets, or ruptures. These conditions may lead to ostomy surgery.

Intestinal obstruction may be either partial or complete. The obstruction could be a paralytic ileus or growths such as tumors or polyps.

Urinary tract malfunctions may result from diseases of the kidney, urethra, ureters, or bladder; neurogenic bladder, exstrophy; accidents; trauma; or cancer.

Congenital anomalies include the following:

1. Myelomeningocele or spina bifida—a congenital defect of the spinal column

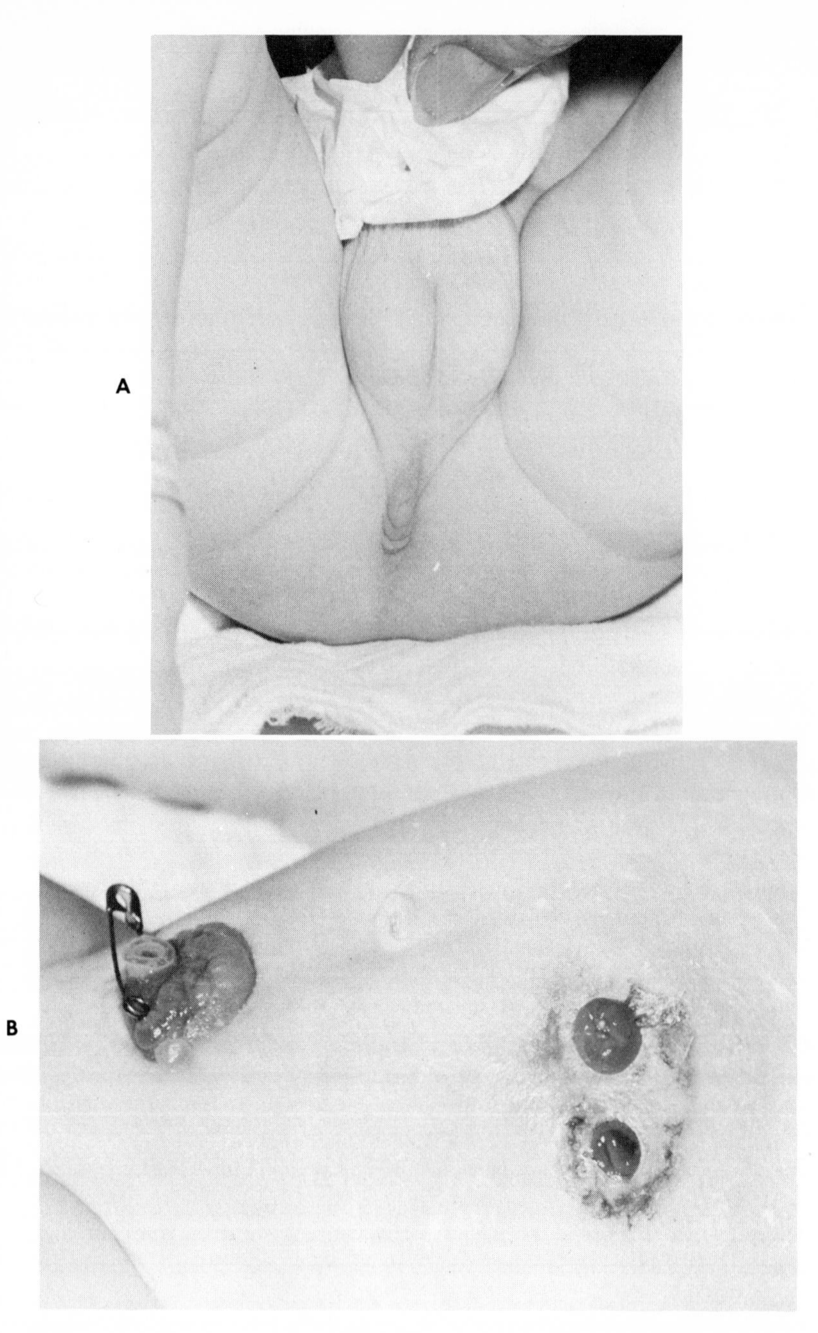

Fig. 4-2. A, Imperforate anus in infant. **B,** Proximal and distal stomas. Splenic flexure of high descending colon and cystostomy of the infant with an imperforate anus.

2. Imperforate anus—an abnormally closed anus at time of birth, which requires surgery for correction
3. Hirschsprung's disease—an abnormal enlargement of a segment of the colon caused by faulty innervation

SURGERY*

The Oxford English Dictionary defines surgery as "the art or practice of treating injuries, deformities and other disorders by manual operation or instrumental appliances."

An 1879 medical dictionary defines surgery as "that branch of the healing art which teaches the proper use of manual operations for the preservation or restoration of health, including such general medicinal and dietetic treatment as the proper performance of such operations may render necessary."

These are definitions of the *word* "surgery." There is no suggestion as to the psychologic or physiologic results of surgery. The patient, the surgeon, and the nurse each have different views on surgery.

Patient. Patients view surgery in relation to personal experience, education, and understanding of the present illness. They are in the very vulnerable position of having to trust the surgeon's judgment that surgery is indicated. They must also have faith in the surgeon's knowledge and skill to perform the surgery, sometimes without what seems to be a satisfactory means of gauging that judgment, knowledge, and skill in advance.

It is normal for persons who are entering surgery to hesitate in entrusting their lives to people they hardly know. Surgery is an invasion of privacy. Intimate knowledge concerning the mental, physical, and often moral lives of patients is written on a chart for surgical and medical personnel to read. When patients have reservations, it is usually because of a misunderstanding or misinterpretation.

Patients fear surgery for various reasons. Some are afraid that it will not correct the problem and they will either die or be required to undergo further surgery. Others fear pain, the unknown, or body changes.

Questions they ask will give the perceptive surgeon or nurse an insight into their fears. They may believe that they have not been told the whole truth, especially if the surgery is estimated as a long or exploratory procedure. Sometimes anxiety is based on surgical experiences of friends or relatives. Most ostomy patients are concerned with body alteration and the fear of social ostracism. Socioeconomic aspects are a major concern also.

Preoperative patient counseling will help to alleviate many of these fears.

Surgeon. The surgeon views surgery as an art and science to be used as a necessary radical means of achieving health. Surgeons also view any surgery as a risk of human life; thus the surgeon must be confident of his training and

---

*From a lecture by Geraldine Ondov, R.N., Education Coordinator and former Operating Room Director, Tucson Medical Center.

skill to ensure the patient a safe operation and conveniently placed stoma that can readily function and facilitate the use of an appliance.

Nurse. The ostomy nurse looks at surgery from a patient care viewpoint, emphasizing the individual's rights to a belief in his dignity and independence. The nurse works with the surgeon to help the patient approach surgery in the best possible health.

It is not uncommon for the surgeon to ask the ostomy nurse for assistance in the operating room during the placement of a Marsan Loop-Loc, a Hollister butterfly bridge, or a temporary pouch. The electrosurgical division of the loop colostomy and the removal of sutures are other procedures with which ostomy nurses may be asked to assist the surgeon.

Sterile pouches

When an established ostomate is admitted to surgery for another reason (e.g., total hip replacement), it is imperative that a sterile field be maintained around the operative site. The ostomy flow, however slight, must be contained during surgery to avoid contamination. Some manufacturers supply sterile pouches in various sizes. If these are not available, pouches may be gas sterilized. The order for a sterile ostomy pouch should be written early enough for the pouch to be sterilized, since the process of sterilization, which includes aeration and culturing, takes time. Most operating rooms or central service departments keep a supply of dated sterile pouches in their supply rooms.

Sterile pouches may also be needed by the surgeon to cover draining fistulas to prevent contamination of the operative site.

TYPES OF OSTOMY SURGERY

Ostomy is performed either as a permanent or a temporary measure, depending on the disease and its complexities. The ostomy is considered permanent when a closure cannot be effected, and temporary until sufficient time has elapsed and the surgeon determines that healthy tissue may be reanastomosed.

Tracheostomy is usually a temporary, small narrow puncture into the windpipe that allows the patient to breathe. Tracheostomy is also the name used for the creation of a permanent opening into the throat of the laryngectomee. This is a large round opening flush with the skin in which the tracheal lumen may be visualized.

*Choledochostomy (*T *tube)* is employed after exploration of the common bile duct or after repair of bile duct stricture. It is a temporary procedure that could last for a period of 6 months.

Esophagostomy is the creation of an artificial opening into the esophagus by transecting the esophagus and bringing the upper part out as a stoma. The lower part of the esophagus is resected as a result of cancer, injuries such as stabs and gunshot wounds, and the swallowing of foreign bodies or caustics

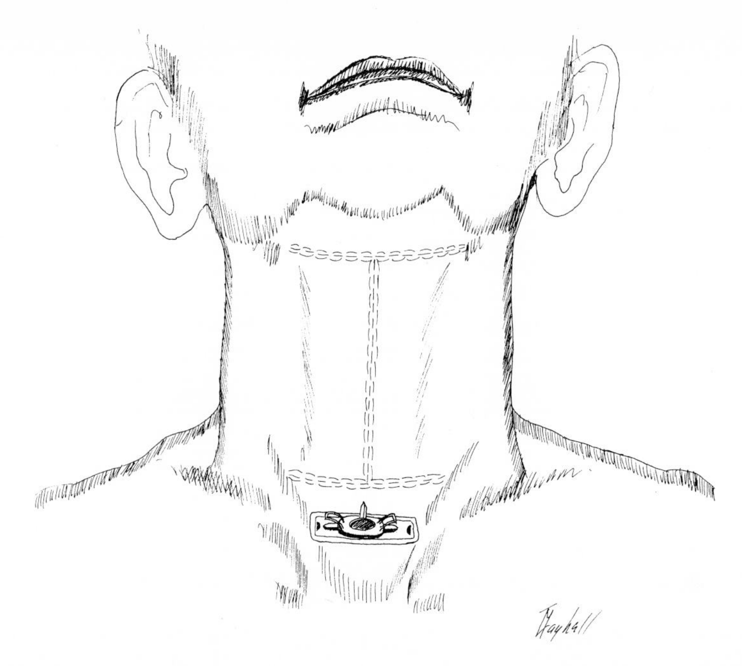

Fig. 4-3. Tracheostomy stoma. (Courtesy Education Department, Tucson Medical Center.)

(strong acids or lye). This procedure allows an egression for oral secretions and provides sufficient time for irradiation of the area resected.

Gastrostomy is an opening into the anterior part of the stomach. It is used for feeding when necessary to maintain adequate nutrition of the patient.

In *jejunostomy* (gastroenterostomy) the jejunum is pulled up and anastomosed with the stomach. A new opening is created, without removal of any portion of the organs, for food to travel from the stomach into the intestines. It is performed for the purpose of feeding through a tube. With the advent of hyperalimentation feedings, this surgery has become less common.

Ileostomy is a surgically created opening of the distal ileum portion of the small intestine through the abdominal wall to the outside, facilitating the elimination of feces. An ileostomy may be established to bypass the entire colon, rectum, and anus. This surgery is primarily performed as a result of ulcerative colitis, familial polyposis, Crohn's disease, injury, or cancer.

Cecostomy is a surgical opening into the cecum. It is usually performed for disease or trauma as a temporary measure to rest the colon. Usually no parts of the colon are removed. If a tube is inserted to relieve colonic obstruction, the surgery is known as a tube cecostomy.

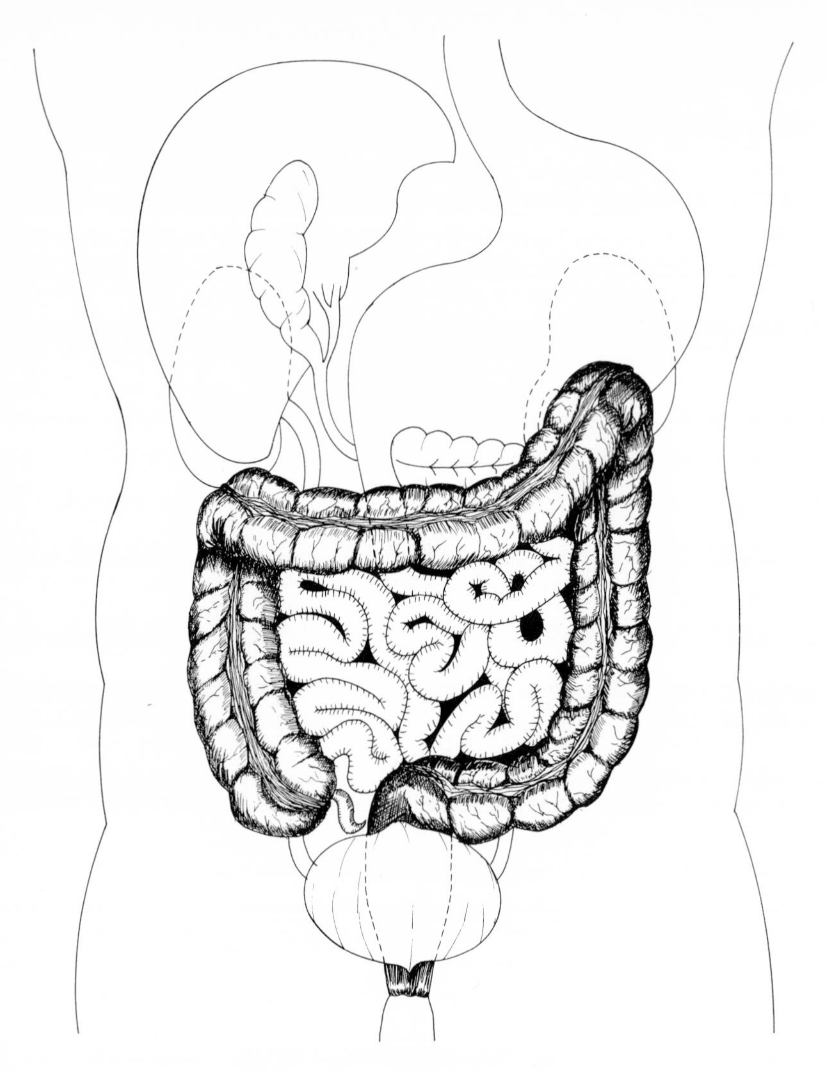

Fig. 4-4. Colon and accessory organs.

In a total *colectomy,* the entire colon is removed and a permanent stoma is established.

Colostomy may be performed on any portion of the large bowel and is predominately performed for malignant growths, diverticulitis, and injury. The tumor mass is removed if the growth has not invaded surrounding viscera. Surgical procedures vary, depending on the growth of the tumor or cancer and the segment involved. Some surgical colostomy procedures are loop, double-barrel, sigmoid, and wet colostomy.

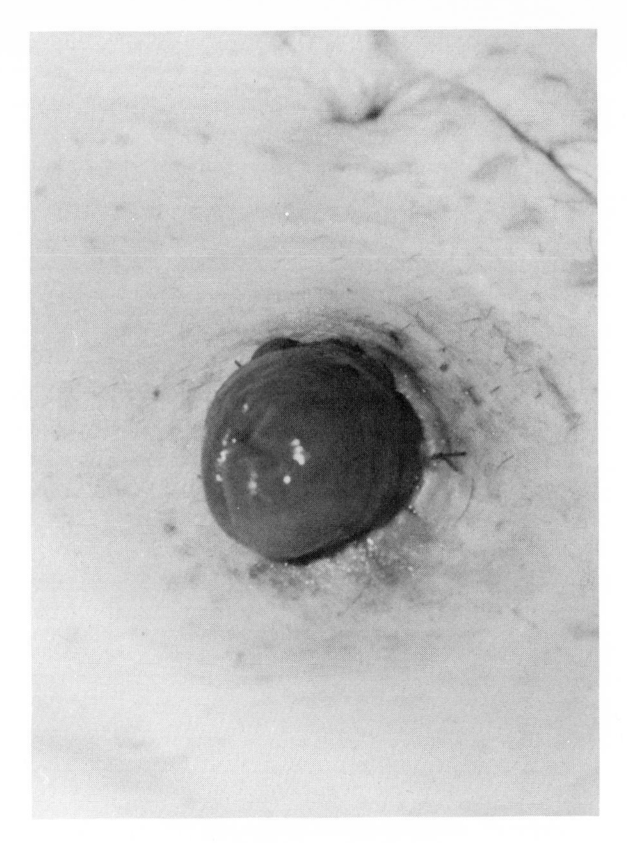

Fig. 4-5. Ileostomy stoma.

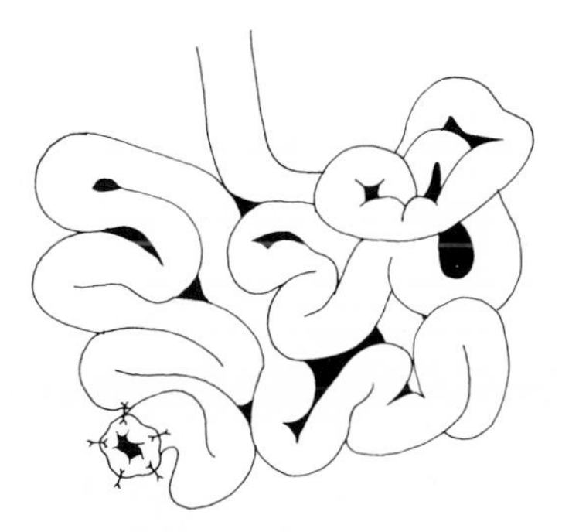

Fig. 4-6. Ileostomy–total colectomy. Colon and rectum have been removed.

The *loop* colostomy (most frequently temporary) is usually performed in the transverse segment to allow the distal part of the colon and/or rectum to heal or rest. A loop of the colon is exteriorized on the abdomen, with a glass or plastic rod placed underneath the intestine for mobilization. Rubber tubing prevents the rod from sliding. The rod is left in place until the bowel becomes adherent to the abdominal wall (approximately 7 days). From 3 to 5 days after surgery, the bowel may be incised laterally to create a single stoma that permits escape of the intestinal contents. Many surgeons prefer to use either the Marsan Loop-Loc appliance or the Hollister Loop Ostomy Bridge instead of the rod and rubber tubing.

The loop is often converted to divided colostomies, usually by electrocautery, forming the *double-barrel* colostomy. The purpose of the division is to facilitate fecal stream diversion until proper healing has occurred and anastomosis is possible. The right-sided or proximal opening is the functioning site, and the left-sided or distal opening is the nonfunctioning mucous fistula.

If the tumor growth is situated in the low *sigmoid* segment, the colon is resected above the growth and a permanent colostomy established. The involved colon with the tumor, rectum, and anus are usually removed.

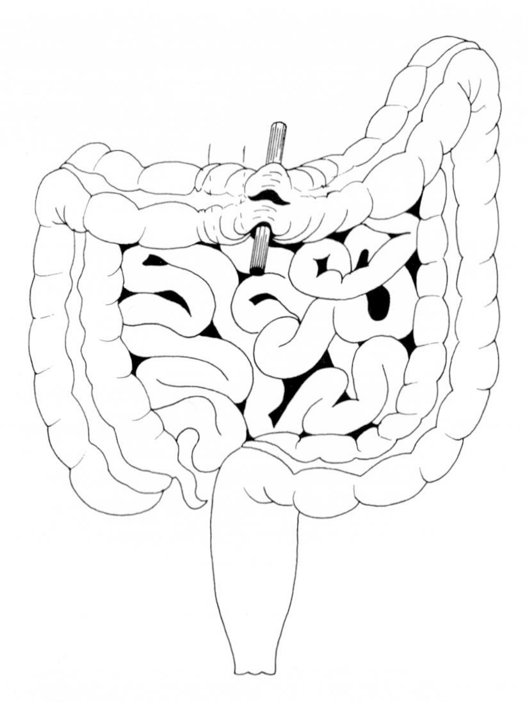

Fig. 4-7. Loop colostomy in transverse colon.

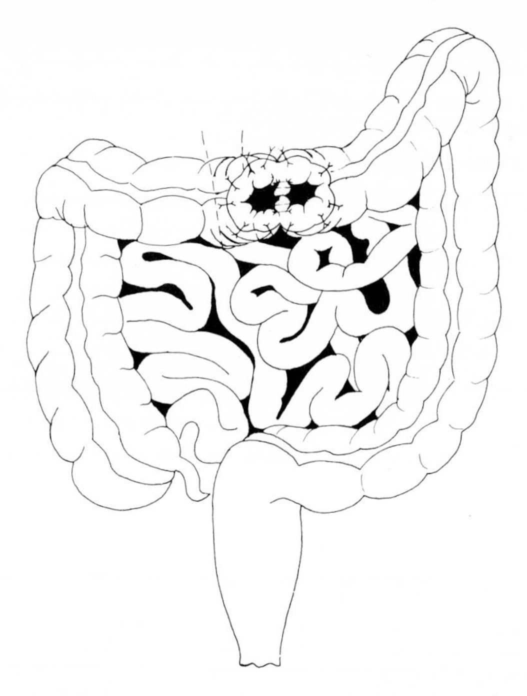

Fig. 4-8. Double-barrel colostomy in transverse colon.

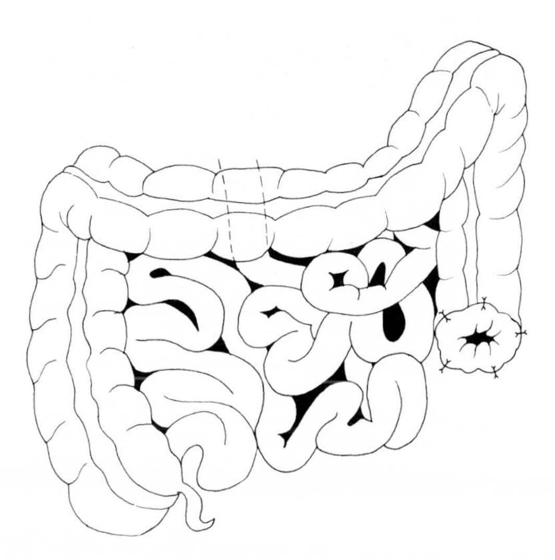

Fig. 4-9. Sigmoid colostomy–abdominoperineal resection. Sigmoid colon and rectum have been removed.

The *wet* colostomy (bilateral ureterosigmoidostomy) is performed to allow excretion of both urine and feces through the stoma. The ureters are resected from the bladder and implanted into the colon. Because of the absorption function of the colon, this procedure is now rarely performed.

Urinary diversions may be performed as a result of loss of the bladder or bladder dysfunction. Surgical openings are provided to allow urinary drainage.

Ileal conduit is often referred to as an ileal bladder because a short segment (approximately 7 inches) of the lower ileum is resected to form a bladder or conduit when restoration of the bladder is not possible. The mesentery of the resected segment remains intact to provide a continual blood supply. The proximal end of the resected ileum section is closed and the distal end is brought through the abdominal wall where a stoma is formed. The ureters, which have been detached from the bladder, are implanted into the conduit

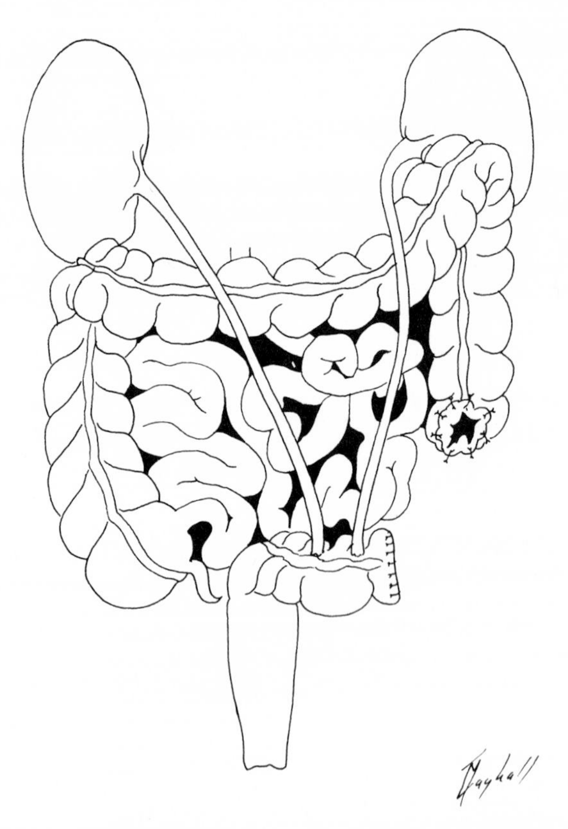

Fig. 4-10. Wet colostomy (bilateral ureterosigmoidostomy). (Courtesy Education Department, Tucson Medical Center.)

for the purpose of draining urine from the kidney to the outside of the body through the stoma on the abdomen. Conditions often requiring ileal conduit surgery are war wounds, abdominal trauma, malignancies that cause destruction or require removal of the bladder, and congenital anomalies.

Cutaneous ureterostomy may be performed when there is stricture or inflammatory obstruction of the ureter. The ureter is detached from the bladder and brought to the abdominal wall, where an opening is made for drainage of

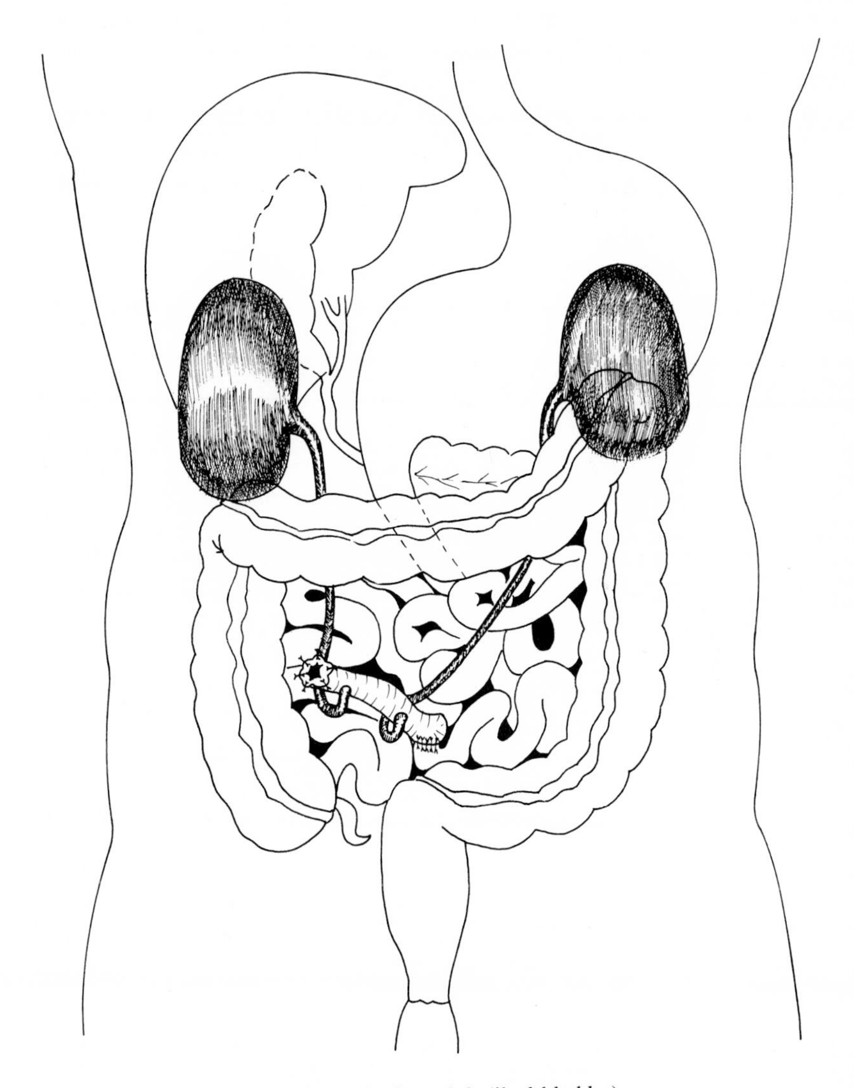

Fig. 4-11. Ileal conduit (ileal bladder).

the ureter. If both ureters are involved, two openings are made. The urine flow is almost constant.

Nephrostomy may be performed for disease, deformity, or obstruction in one or both kidneys. A permanent or temporary opening (depending on the involvement) is made on the posterior section of the body at waist level into the pelvis of the kidney. The urine drains directly from the kidney to the outside through a catheter.

Vesicostomy is usually for trauma or deformity. Generally no parts are removed. The bladder is brought forward and sutured to the abdominal wall, and an opening is made through the abdominal wall into the bladder to permit urine elimination.

Pelvic exenteration is indicated when a neoplasm, which does not tend to metastasize and is confined in a pelvic viscus, has been proved incurable by a lesser operation or radiation therapy. The patient's age, general physical condition, and ability to cope with the radical surgery should be major considerations.

Complete or total exenteration necessitates both fecal and urinary diversion. The surgical procedure consists of an en bloc removal of the rectum, distal sigmoid colon, urinary bladder and distal ureters, internal iliac vessels and their lateral branches, and all pelvic reproductive organs and lymph node. Female total exenteration also includes excision of the entire pelvic floor with accompanying pelvic peritoneum levator muscles and perineum.

Ileal pouch (also called the Kock procedure,* continent ileostomy, or intra-abdominal intestinal reservoir) is still in the experimental stage and not recommended for all ileostomy candidates. Approximately 40 cm (16 inches) of terminal ileum are used in the procedure.The pouch is constructed from 30 cm and the remaining portion is utilized for the nipple valve inside the pouch and an abdominal stoma. The intestinal content of the reservoir (pouch) is evacuated through a catheter that has been inserted into the stoma and through the valve.

---

*Nils G. Kock, Department of Surgery, Sahlgren's Hospital, University of Göteborg, Sweden.

CHAPTER 5

Counseling program

Counseling is the interchange of opinions or instructions, given on request or deliberation, for directing the judgment or conduct of another. It is used in many ways. Professional practitioners use counseling as a therapeutic tool by utilizing psychologic principles to guide the individual to a better understanding of his problems and potentialities. Patients undergoing ostomy surgery have particular anxieties and needs. Counseling the ostomy candidate helps alleviate these anxieties and enhances emotional stability. Several sessions may be required as the patient is guided through the duration of his hospital stay. Counseling could continue after his discharge through telephone calls, home visits, or a return to the stoma clinic.

Medical centers today are recognizing that the ostomy nurse, who is conversant with ostomy problems, can, without appearing overoptimistic or unnecessarily casual, build a picture of health and optimism for the patient to ensure his transition from surgery through his convalescence.

FOURFOLD INVOLVEMENT

The involvement of the ostomy nurse in counseling is fourfold because an effective relationship among the physician, patient, family, and nursing staff is best maintained through a counseling process.

The *physician* must order patient counseling and determine what degree and type of information the patient is to receive. The knowledge the *patient* receives before surgery helps him through the first week without apprehension and contributes to successful recuperation. Postoperative counseling prepares the patient for going home, hopefully with the ability to cope with the aspects of ostomy management. The *family* is included in counseling as an aid in the continuous emotional support of the patient. *Nursing personnel* are vital to the patient's physical and emotional transition from illness to health and must be involved in the counseling process to enhance their knowledge of the ostomy patient.

Counseling may be initiated before the patient is admitted to the hospital or after he is an established ostomate. In most cases the program outlined here may be adapted to the individual needs of the patient and those involved with him.

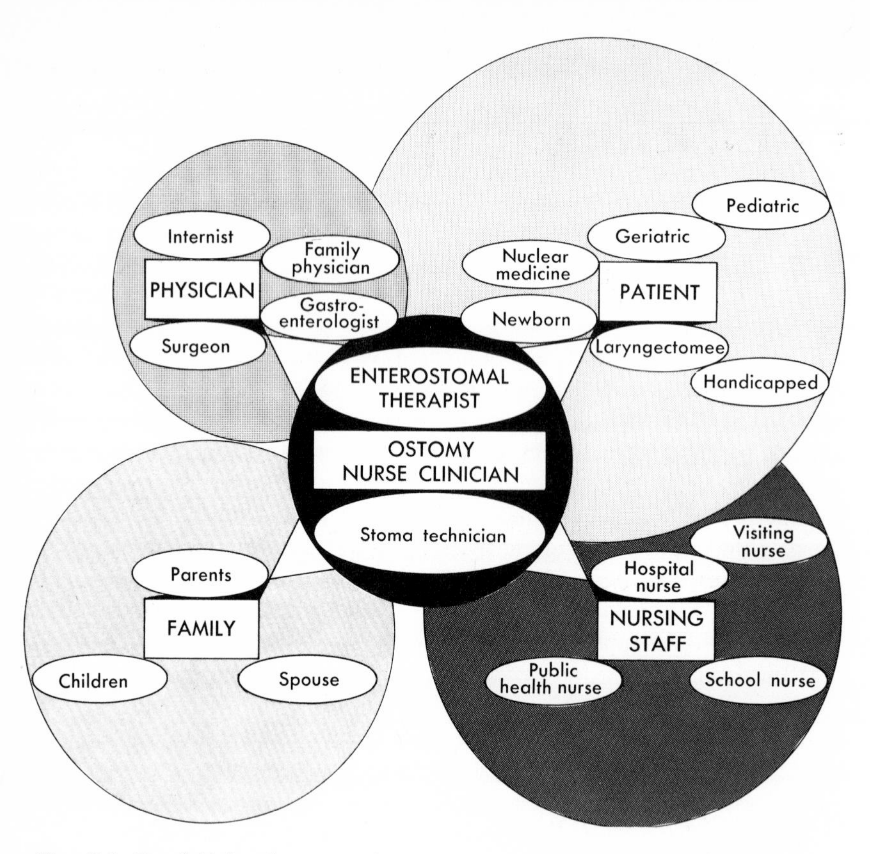

Fig. 5-1. Fourfold involvement of the ostomy nurse with the patient, physician, family, and nurse.

Patient

The first counseling session is usually scheduled according to the physician's order, but subsequent sessions may be at opportune times, as indicated. Sufficient time must be alloted for the patient to express his fears, facilitating a better understanding of the immediate vital change. One hour should be ample time for a relaxed question and answer session. Since the patient has a right to privacy, quiet, comfortable surroundings should be selected for this session. The ostomy nurse talks casually with the patient while mentally evaluating his responses or attitudes regarding his present illness. The knowledge the patient possesses serves as a good basis for the continued interview.

An anatomic chart will be an asset in promoting the patient's understanding of his forthcoming surgery. As the patient visualizes where his surgical opening will be, the ostomy nurse may explain the meaning of the word "stoma" and discuss permanent and temporary ostomies.

A stoma pouch placed on the patient's abdomen at the proposed stoma site, filled with 10 ml of water, and worn by the patient for 24 hours will give him a realistic idea of body management.

Since ostomy surgeries vary, some patients may require specifics that do not apply to other ostomates.

Laryngectomee. This patient will need to understand that immediately after surgery he will be unable to talk. He will breathe by means of a tube in the trachea and will be fed intravenously or through a temporary tube that has been inserted in the nostril. Postoperatively, the patient should learn to care for his stoma and to develop new methods of communication. A hand-operated mechanical device held to the laryngectomee's neck permits him to communicate, but most patients prefer to learn esophageal speech. This is a method by which air is taken into the esophagus and expelled through the mouth. A local club member of the International Association of Laryngectomees (IAL) and the speech therapist are valuable allies in counseling this patient.

Geriatric patient. The actual age of the geriatric patient is not the main concern when counseling the patient. A young 80-year-old may have a morbid fear of dependency on others and feel a loss of self-esteem, while an old 60-year-old may demand that someone assume responsibility for his complete care and will reject counseling. The spouse is a valuable asset to the geriatric patient, but if the patient is alone or if the family has no facilities for patient care, a medicenter or extended nursing care facility may be the answer until he can care for himself. This should be discussed with the patient and his family during a counseling session.

Patients with a language barrier. A language barrier is frightening to all patients. Their fear of being left alone is very real, and the fact that they are unable to communicate specific needs is very frustrating to them. Some communication can be effected by a touch or a look, and with skilled instruction the patient can be taught to care for his own body and appliance. However, most hospitals have personnel in their employ who are familiar with languages and who can serve as interpreters when necessary. A list of these employees may be kept convenient to all staff.

Handicapped persons. The ostomy itself is not a handicap, but some patients who have ostomies are otherwise handicapped. Arthritic individuals, the blind, amputees, and those with loss of function from stroke or spinal cord injury will need special information to enable them to cope with the body change.

Where these special problems exist, the major concern is to place the stoma where it may be reached and cared for with ease. The appliance is also an important consideration. A one-piece appliance promotes confidence and allows more ease in handling and changing. The blind ostomate can learn to care for his body and perfect the appliance change just as he can learn to read in braille, cook, or eat. The handicapped patient may require more counseling to accept the fact that another inconvenience has been added.

Patients receiving nuclear medicine treatment. With the development of new scientific devices and techniques, radiation therapy is now used in treating certain ostomy patients. The alert nurse recognizes the need for understanding the clinical uses of radiation and the special patient involved. Nuclear medicine procedures and precautions are clearly explained to the patient by the radiologist, and the nurse will be required to follow specific written procedures.

Newborn. Parents of an infant ostomy candidate need special counseling, since it is difficult for parents to accept the fact that their newborn child must undergo this serious operation. They will need to be taught how to care for the child's ostomy in whatever manner is most convenient. Most infant ostomies are temporary and are later closed. Permanent surgeries will be followed through the growing years until the child has gained independence in self-care.

Pediatric patients. Counseling for the child must be commensurate with his age and understanding. The older child may be counseled several weeks before surgery, enabling him to cope with his fears. He will repeat the same questions many times, seeking reassurance.

The younger child will not understand or have as many questions; therefore 1 or 2 weeks prior to surgery is ample time for the child to be counseled.

Some children may be too ill or unable to grasp the idea of surgery and its meaning, but those who are receptive should understand that ostomy surgery is the remedy for their discomfort. More pediatric counseling is necessary when the child finally sees the result of the surgery. Counseling will acqaint him with the fact that he is no longer ill and can participate in school activities, sports, and daily living.

The pediatric ostomate should learn to assume responsibility for his ostomy care. Even the small child can assist until he is old enough to be taught to care for himself. One of the dominant considerations in the care of any ostomy patient is cleanliness. This is particularly important with the pediatric patient and should be stressed. If the child is aware that cleanliness makes him feel better, heal faster, and be more acceptable to his family and friends, he will strive for cleanliness. Overprotection encourages dependency and should be avoided.

Family

Including the spouse or the patient's family in counseling sessions often eliminates confusion and the need for repetition and offers more support to the patient because he can discuss the situtation with his family. The anxieties of the family are easily transmitted to the patient and may slow his progress. Family counseling promotes mutual understanding and reduces these anxieties.

Spouse. An understanding spouse is an invaluable aid to alleviating apprehension in the ostomy patient. The ostomy nurse may counsel the spouse in additional sessions separately from the mate. Reassurance is often extended to the spouse by extra counseling while the patient is in the operating room; this is a time that easily lends itself to questions and answers of particular concern.

Parents. It is natural for parents to feel stress as they learn that their child must undergo ostomy surgery. The manner in which the parents cope with this stress situation greatly influences the child's acceptance or denial of his altered body image.

Unprepared parents may experience an enormous shock as they contemplate the results of ostomy surgery on their child. When parents have sufficient time to learn as much as possible about the proposed surgery and discuss their fears with parents of young ostomates, they will more readily accept the idea of their own child's surgery. The counselor will assure the parents that unless other problems are involved, after recovery and adjustment the child may again participate in sports, be able to marry, and have children. The child's anticipated sexual development may be discussed with the surgeon or the nurse at puberty.

One or both parents should be present several times for appliance change and cleaning of the stoma area to gain an understanding of the mechanics involved in adapting and individualizing a particular technique for the child.

Children or siblings of ostomates. All children in a family will be involved when a member of that family is scheduled for ostomy surgery and will need counseling. To facilitate freedom of expression, counseling sessions should be held when the ill family member is absent.

To accommodate the new surgical patient, either a parent or a sibling, family routine will probably require change. After the patient has recovered from his surgery and his living habits have been established, the children should easily adapt to the new routine. As understanding evolves and as health returns, the new ostomate is absorbed into the normal daily family life. Except for appliance change, there is no way to tell which one has the ostomy.

Nursing staff

Staff nurse. An educational program in ostomy care will facilitate the expansion of nursing actions to prevent, minimize, or alleviate problems for the ostomy patient.

School nurse. The ostomy nurse or the parents should have a private counseling session with the school nurse when a child has recovered from ostomy surgery and must return to daily school activities. An understanding school nurse will arrange timely bathroom privileges for the student. If the student participates in a physical education program, private shower time may be planned. The college student can enjoy dormitory living if proper provisions have been previously arranged.

Industrial or occupational nurse. Industrial companies employ one or more nurses who are responsible for the health services of the company. They are interested mainly in keeping employees well and on the job but often serve as counselors or advisors.

The industrial nurse can be valuable to the ostomate in the readjustment period that occurs when the ostomate returns to work after his recovery from the surgery.

Public health or community nurse. Public health or community nurses visit patients in their homes, at work, or at school and act as health consultants. They are often the vital link between the patient and public resources, since they work closely with hospitals and other agencies.

Visiting nurse. Visiting nurses usually establish treatment protocols with the physician and the ostomy nurse before the patient is discharged. They are able to monitor the patient's home care and coordinate with physicians the patient's independence or plans for long-term care. Visiting nurses may reduce the trips the patient makes to the physician's office or clinic.

FACING SOCIETY

The patient no sooner becomes adjusted to the hospital setting than he must face the idea of an adjustment to society. Being discharged is both an exciting and an anxious event, but with planning, this becomes another phase of progress. Returning to the job, school, or society follows normally when the patient is prepared.

PSYCHOSEXUAL ASPECTS

The successful return to a sexual relationship maintained by the ostomate prior to surgery is influenced by the emotional attitude of the patient toward the physical changes in his body. Surveys conducted on the psychosexual adjustment of ostomates indicate that the eventual return of the patient to a normal position in his family is predicated on several factors:

1. The basic psychosexual attitude of the patient
2. The illness and its accompanying psychologic and physiologic changes, which make the patient more concerned with survival than sexual matters
3. The postoperative period, when the patient is learning the functions and care of the stoma
4. The readjustment period, when the ostomate's progress is relative to his own abilities and attitudes

A psychologic dilemma exists to some degree in all ostomy patients. The preoperative physical and mental status of the patient will influence his postoperative adjustment. Well-adjusted patients will adapt more favorably to the change in their self-image. Patients with physiologic or psychosexual problems before the illness will in all probability continue to be influenced by these problems after surgery.

The readjustment period for a patient who has undergone emergency surgery may be more difficult, since the patient has not had time to prepare himself for the change in his physical conditon. In either case, the spouse's reaction is a major factor in determining the patient's progress in returning to normal interpersonal and sexual relationships. Visits with other ostomy patients may also help the patient reestablish confidence in himself.

A common fear among male patients is that the surgery may interfere with sexual relationships. Surveys have shown that only 15% of male ostomates experience a decrease in sexual activity. If nerve damage is not evident, lack of sexual function is most probably psychologic.

Fear of not being able to conceive a child is a natural concern of the female ostomy patient. It has been found that there is less incidence of nerve damage in the female because of her wider pelvic structure, making the female's readjustment to normal sexual activity easier than the male's.

Obstetricians have reported that ostomy surgery does not necessarily interfere with conception, pregnancy, or delivery of a healthy child. Also, pregnancy seldom produces complications in the care and proper functioning of the stoma. Regular checkups, proper diet, and sufficient exercise are the same as those prescribed for other expectant mothers. Many physicians recommend that ostomy patients delay pregnancy for 1 to 2 years after surgery. Delivery may be by cesarean section, but this is no more common in ostomy patients than in others. Episiotomy, which is performed in a large percentage of women, is usually necessary in any ostomy patient if the rectum has been excised.

Marriage need not be prohibited for male or female ostomates. It should be pointed out, however, that ostomy patients must first return to normal interpersonal relationships and overcome their feelings of physical incompetence. Once they know they are socially accepted, the return to normal sexual relationships will follow naturally.

TRAVEL*

The ostomy counseling program should include travel information. Suggestions from experienced ostomate travelers are listed here.

1. *Identification.* Carry an identification card with information concerning the type of ostomy, whether irrigation is necessary, and other pertinent information.
2. *Ostomy supplies.* Plan to take an excess of supplies. Keep a change available at all times. Other accessories include plastic bags for disposable purposes, toilet tissue, towelettes, water for irrigating, a large bath towel, and thumbtacks for use in public restrooms without privacy considerations.

---

*From a lecture by Hilde Dahne, member of the Mission Ostomy Association, Tucson, and formerly of Jodan Tours of Tokyo.

3. *Medications.* Carry medications that are properly identified. The physician should be contacted for additional prescriptions that might be needed during travel.
4. *Self-contained camper.* The camper is not unlike home-living conditions. Make any change in routine as slight as possible. Take along bottled water or drinking water from home. In many states, bottled water is available in vending machines.
5. *Car travel*
   a. If possible, carry a cooler for juices or special food needs.
   b. Eat as little as possible.
   c. When eating at restaurants, avoid the unusual, exotic, or buffet foods that have been unrefrigerated for more than an hour. Eat at large restaurants that offer a variety of selections.
   d. Place the seat belt above or below the stoma to avoid pressure.
6. *Diarrhea.* If medications are unsuccessful in preventing or controlling diarrhea, try pure chocolate (not candy bars). Do not allow diarrhea to continue; see a physician.
7. *Air travel*
   a. Arrange for private inspection of carry-on luggage in advance if desired.
   b. Appliances with metal parts may cause a security alarm problem. Show the guard an extra appliance to alleviate this problem.
   c. Check through only extra supplies with the luggage. Carry a tote bag with regular supplies onto the plane.
   d. Important: remove air from medication tubes or droppers. Remove caps, apply gentle pressure to the tube, expel the air, and then replace the caps.
   e. Either ask in advance about food that is served on the airplane, carry food in the tote bag, or, if in doubt, do not eat.
8. *International travel*
   a. Inform the tour guide in advance concerning special considerations such as an understanding roommate. Private rooms are usually available, but they are more expensive. The tour guide will also assist in the customs inspection.
   b. When traveling, plan sightseeing trips around personal care time.
   c. Carry a personal supply kit at all times.
   d. As a precaution, prepare a list of clinics, physicians, hospitals, and ostomy associations that may be contacted during the tour. Assistance lists are obtainable from the United Ostomy Association, Los Angeles, California, or the International Association of Medical Assistance to Travelers (IAMAT), Suite 5620, 350 Fifth Avenue, New York, N.Y. American Military or mission hospitals as well as the American embassies are available to tourists.

e. Do not drink tap water or water in thermos jars that are supplied by hotels. Ask for bottled water with unbroken seals. A small amount of water can do a great deal of harm. Pure water must be used for irrigations as well as drinking. Water purifiers are available for emergency situations.
f. Do not drink soft drinks internationally. American brand names on the drinks are no indication that they have been "made in America." Local water combined with sugar provides a perfect medium for bacterial growth.
g. Eat well-cooked foods. Wash unpeeled fresh foods and peel them. If the skin is broken on the food, discard it. It is best not to take a chance on uncooked foods.
h. Buy canned junior foods available in gourmet departments of large markets.
i. Avoid cream pastries, another good medium for bacterial growth.
j. Use good judgment in selecting places where meats are served. Meats in other countries may not be subjected to the strict inspection laws of the United States.
k. Adjust colostomy irrigation time according to the various time zones.

EVALUATING THE SESSIONS

The ostomy nurse interprets and evaluates the substance of each counseling session. Evaluation is both general and specific. General evaluations present the patient's overall strengths and weaknesses, disabilities and potentialities. A specific evaluation identifies individual problems and any situations influencing a particular problem.

CHAPTER 6

Preoperative care

The degree or intensity of preoperative preparation is planned in proportion to the ramifications of the surgery. The patient scheduled for an ostomy procedure should be admitted to the hospital 2 or 3 days prior to surgery.

It is important that the patient understand that ostomy surgery is the end of a complex health problem and that the next step is recovery. Physiologic and psychologic counseling are important preoperatively as well as postoperatively.

The ostomy nurse's initial contact with a patient usually occurs soon after hospital admission. This serves to introduce the nurse to the patient and possibly the family. Supportive communication alleviates a degree of anxiety and uncertainty and often motivates patient participation in the preoperative preparation.

Communicating with someone other than the family frequently creates a more positive acceptance of the pending surgery. For this reason the physician may request a preoperative visit from a visitor trained by the American Cancer Society or the United Ostomy Association.

Candidates for surgery frequently suffer from serious malnutrition. This is especially true of chronically ill patients. Nutritional deficiencies must be assessed and corrected.

BOWEL PREPARATION

The most important principle common to gastrointestinal surgeries is to operate on an empty tract and to keep it empty during the early postoperative recovery period. In elective surgeries, the physician may instruct patients to begin a preoperative diet regimen at home, consisting of an approximately 3-day oral bulk-free chemical diet. Bowel preparation supports the nutritional needs of patients and enhances body healing ability by promoting a positive nitrogen balance.

The preparation of the bowel by an elemental diet has now been documented in medical journals and is being employed by many surgeons.

The ostomy nurse or the surgeon should counsel patients concerning the advantages of using the elemental diet method for bowel preparation. The unpalatable aspects of the diet are sometimes difficult for patients to accept. The soluble powder may be mixed with juice or ginger ale and frozen into slushes or sickles to make it more palatable.

Formulas are individualized to the specific needs and conditions of patients.

Indications for total elemental alimentation

1. Patients depleted of protein reserves resulting from disease of the gastrointestinal tract
   a. Ulcerative colitis, acute
   b. Granulomatous disease of the small and large bowel
   c. Chronic infection
   d. Cancer of the stomach or colon, preoperative preparation
   e. Malabsorption syndrome
   f. Chronic malnutrition of various types
2. Patients with partial function of the gastrointestinal tract
   a. Esophageal, gastric, and duodenal fistulas with feeding distal to the fistula
   b. Small bowel fistulas with feeding either proximal or distal, depending on the level
   c. Colonic fistula (low bulk)
   d. Short gut syndrome
3. Nutritional preparation prior to radiologic examination or surgery
   a. Preoperative bowel preparation to avoid semistarvation or excessive catharsis

Three-day method utilizing Vivonex-HN (high nitrogen)

Day 1 Clear liquid diet
Vivonex-HN (3 packs)
60 ml milk of magnesia with orange juice twice a day

Day 2 Clear liquid diet
Vivonex-HN (3 packs)
60 ml milk of magnesia with orange juice twice a day
Tap water enemas until clear in the morning and evening

Day 3 Clear liquid diet
Vivonex-HN (3 packs)
60 ml milk of magnesia with orange juice twice a day
Tap water enemas until clear in the morning and evening

Mixing Vivonex-HN (powdered form)

1. Place one package of Vivonex powder in a bowl.
2. Slowly add 12 ounces of cold water, beating constantly.
3. Continue beating until the solution is smooth.
4. Chill the glass in a freezer 1 hour prior to use.
5. Pour the solution into the chilled glass.
6. Place the glass in a small container of chipped ice to keep it chilled if

frosting in the freezer does not keep the glass cold during sipping. (The glass should remain chilled while the patient sips the liquid.)

7. Instructions to the patient
   a. Place the straw well back in the mouth. Avoid contact with all taste buds.
   b. Slowly sip the liquid. Slow sipping allows the colon to absorb all the liquid. The patient may wish to listen to music, watch television, or read while ingesting the formula.
   c. After the glass has been emptied, bite on a slice of orange, lime, or lemon to remove any unpleasant taste.

NASOGASTRIC TUBE

Before surgery, the nasogastric tube is inserted through the nostril into the stomach to aid in decompression. When the patient understands that his cooperation is required to promote the smooth insertion of the nasogastric tube, he will more readily accept instructions to swallow as the tube goes down.

DEEP BREATHING

Deep breathing is important to the patient, aiding in lung expansion and stimulating blood flow to the lungs. The patient should be aware that chest breathing is only moving the chest, while deep breathing involves the mid-abdomen. The patient's hand is placed on his diaphragm and he is asked to inhale until he feels the movement of the breathing process.

EXERCISES

Exercises may be used to prevent the body from becoming static. Movement of the wrists and ankles is easy for the patient to accomplish and particularly useful until he is ready for ambulation. A method of rotating the ankles and wrists should be demonstrated, and the patient should know that he is helping himself by doing these exercises regularly during waking periods.

SPIRITUAL THERAPY*

Spiritual therapy is as important to some patients as medication. "Man is by constitution a religious being."† Spiritual aspects lend purpose and meaning to human existence. Individuals often feel a greater need for spiritual help during an illness, especially those who are terminally ill or facing surgery.

Patients entering the hospital bring their religious beliefs, and often religious articles, with them. Emotional and mental reactions have a definite effect on physical health, and supporting these beliefs promotes peace of mind

---

*Based on sermon notes from the late Reverend E. L. Douglass.

†From Spencer, Herbert: Principles of sociology, Vol. III, New York, N.Y., 1898.

and healing. Many people who profess to have no faith will ask for spiritual aid when sickness or death approaches them or a loved one.

Surgery is a time of crisis. Regardless of how prepared individuals may be, they usually have doubts and fears of the unknown and the possibility of death. These fears and doubts can only be helped by religious sources. Some patients have an attitude against any type of religion, and their beliefs must be respected.

Requests for spiritual help must originate with patients. It is important for nurses to be as aware of patients' desires for *no* religious counseling as it is to recognize signs from patients who want to ask for assurance but are too shy or embarrassed. A flippant answer such as "See you later," may be a plea for assurance that they really will be there later.

Clergy can be valuable members of the health team, since they have a background of experience in helping persons who are going through difficult times. They are involved listeners who demonstrate trust. There are no magic words that will erase all fears, but patients can be helped to face some realities. Patients and families may be able to verbalize their fears more readily with the clergy.

Hospital chaplains administer spiritual support on a nondenominational basis. Individual religious preference is indicated on hospital admission sheets, and most hospitals have a procedure for contacting clergy.

Ostomy nurses may feel no personal involvement in spiritual matters, but they should be prepared to handle situations that might arise. Through counseling or self-care teaching sessions, nurses establish rapport with patients who may feel that ostomy nurses can help them with a spiritual problem. Patients' spiritual patterns are as important as their breathing patterns, and nurses should be alert to these needs. If adequate answers cannot be given by them, nurses should seek the proper clerical assistance.

MARKING THE STOMA SITE

Placement of the stoma is an important preoperative consideration. The method used to mark the abdomen must be approved by the surgeon. To assess wearing ability of the appliance, a disk and pouch may be placed on the patient's abdomen. Existing scars and bony prominences must be avoided if the appliance is to fit properly. The disk and pouch are removed, and the stoma site may be marked with 10% brilliant green (specially constituted in the pharmacy). This preparation will remain after the skin has been prepared for surgery. Some surgeons recommend using a coin (nickel) to obtain the correct circumference. Instead of marking the site with green, some surgeons may prefer that the stoma site be nicked for better identification.

PREOPERATIVE VISIT BY THE OPERATING ROOM NURSE

Many hospitals have initiated an operating room nurse preoperative visitation program. Patients who are scheduled for afternoon surgery are visited in the morning; those scheduled for morning surgery are visited the preceding afternoon or evening.

Subjects discussed include the shave prep, changing into the hospital gown, administration of the preoperative medication, the surgery suite, the surgical team, the anesthesiologist, the surgical lights, and the recovery room.

CHAPTER 7

Postoperative care

On returning to consciousness, the patient may express concern about the outcome of the operation. He should be reassured with brief, appropriate information that the surgery is over. The nursing staff is concerned with the postoperative care of the patient.

Body comfort

1. Encourage deep breathing.
2. Promote mouth care by rinsing the mouth with antiseptics.
3. Apply alcohol or soothing lotion to the patient's back and stroke gently.
4. Place a small pillow in the hollow of the patient's back to alleviate tiredness.
5. Turn the patient frequently.

Observation

1. Surgical dressings for any signs of bleeding
2. Collection pouches for output
3. Intravenous fluids for electrolyte imbalance
4. Body temperature
5. Postoperative fluids, to meet electrolyte and nutritional needs of the patient
6. Intake and output recordings
7. Drainage or clotting
8. Drug reaction
9. Any purulent drainage or signs of infection

To prevent cross infection of patients or personnel, there should always be an emphasis placed on handwashing.

OSTOMY PATIENTS REQUIRING SPECIAL PROCEDURES

Some ostomy patients will require special procedures according to the surgery performed.

Laryngostomy

The laryngostomy patient usually has postoperative depression, which is normal, because he is alarmed when he cannot speak. Since early attempts to speak must be avoided, writing materials should be provided for the patient's convenience in communication.

Since a patent airway is necessary to maintain life, it is important that the laryngectomee be suctioned nasally as well as tracheally because he can no longer blow his nose. The suctioning should be gentle but firm, using the Y connector instead of a straight connector.

Elevating the head of the bed 30 to 45 degrees will help the patient's breathing and lessen tension on his sutures. The patient's head and neck should be supported when his position is changed.

The nasogastric tube will probably remain fixed from 7 to 10 days, and the area around the tube must be kept clean. Fluids should be administered at room temperature to avoid nausea and abdominal cramps.

Tracheostomy

Tracheostomy care should be performed every 4 hours and more often if necessary. The tracheostomy opening and skin should be washed with hydrogen peroxide or a nondetergent soap to clean the stoma area. Redness of this area should be called to the attention of the physician. Cultures of tracheal secretions, taken weekly, allow early detection of possible infection.

The tracheal tube is held in place by tapes fastened around the patient's neck. It is important that the tracheostomy be kept open, and moist air is necessary to prevent mucous plugs.

Gastrostomy

The nasogastric tube is usually left in place several days postoperatively. The excessive secretions should be removed from around the nostrils, and if the patient breathes through his mouth, it should be kept well oiled and rinsed. Pressure of the tube on the nostrils can be avoided by fixing the tube under the nose. To fix the tube, the skin should first be prepared with benzoin and/or skin prep. A small strip of nonallergic tape is placed on the prepared skin and the tube positioned over the tape and anchored with a second piece of tape.

Urinary diversion

Indwelling catheters should be kept aseptic. Cultures should be taken when signs of infection are indicated. The best specimen is obtained from the ileal conduit by inserting a cathether 2 inches into the conduit.

Abdominal-perineal resection

Abdominal-perineal resection is usually performed when an ileostomy or sigmoid colostomy is necessary. Frequently, the rectal defect will have a sump tube in place. A sterile peri-pad may be necessary for a few days. When the patient is ambulatory, a sitz bath followed by the use of a perineal lamp for 10 minutes often promotes healing of the suture line and adds to the patient's comfort. If healing by first intention is slow and drainage continues, a biweekly instillation of neomycin suspension, usually 1% strength, may hasten the healing time and decrease drainage.

Perineal wounds

The perineal wound refers to the space left after the rectum has been removed. This area of the body does not have a particularly good blood supply, which is important to satisfactory healing; frequently, fistulas or abscesses will occur if the skin surface of the wound closes first. It is important that the space left after the removal of the rectum heal by first intention (from within outward) and that the skin opening be the last to close. This will result in a firm healing of the wound with no spaces left where fluid can accumulate and become infected.

Perineal wound healing time varies with the individual. It could occur within a period of several months to many years. There must be strict adherence to a program of local hygiene whereby the area is kept clean and free from infection, thus, allowing the body's healing defenses time to work.

The ostomy nurse may institute a perineal care procedure for the inpatient and teach the patient a self-care adaptation of the procedure before he is discharged.

Procedure for perineal wound care. The procedure for perineal care is a synthesis of related nursing care interventions: catheter care, both rectal and bladder if indicated; cleansing of the anal site; irrigation of the rectal defect and employment of prescriptions; sitz bath, chair or tub; and lamping.

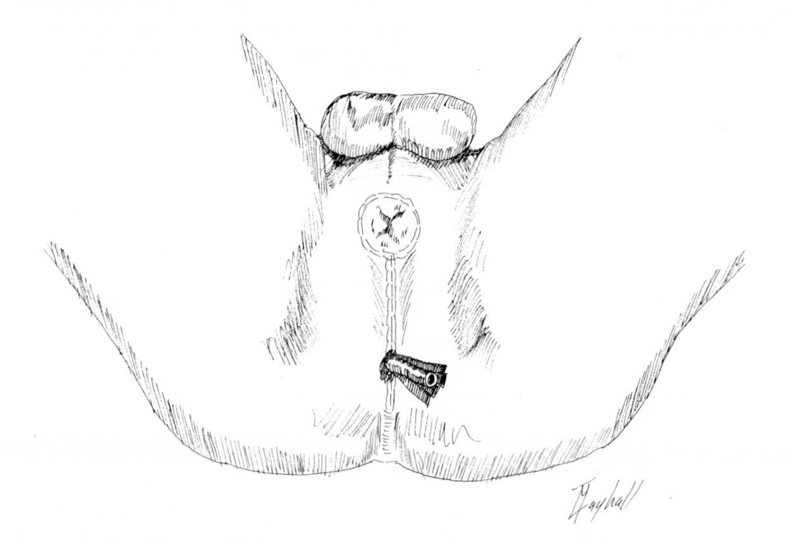

Fig. 7-1. Rectal drainage. (Courtesy Education Department, Tucson Medical Center.)

The following procedure incorporates these interventions.

Purpose. To clean the perineum of the patient who has had any type of colorectal surgery, or surgery involving this area where drainage occurs, to prevent infection, to enhance healing, to relieve the patient of irritation and discomfort, to relieve retention of urine, and to promote drainage of the rectal defect.

Equipment for full procedure

Peri-care tray consisting of a covered pitcher, sterile cotton balls, forceps and holder, towels, and wash cloth
Cleansing solution (as preferred or ordered by the physician)
Tap water (90° to 100° F) or medicated solution (as ordered by the physician)
Bedpan and cover
Plastic square and plastic bag
Peri-pads and ABD pads
Bath blanket
Bath thermometer
Ointment (if ordered by the physician)
Sterile applicators for applying the ointment
Irrigating catheter for irrigating the rectal defect (eg, Bard No. 18)
50 ml syringe for irrigation
Sitz bath, chair or tub
  Bath mat
  Slippers for the patient
  Glass of juice for the patient to sip
  Water 105° to 110° F
Lamp with a 60-watt bulb

Specific procedures

For cleansing the perineum

1. Wash hands.
2. Explain the procedure to the patient. Any time a procedure is introduced for the first time, an explanation may help the patient to accept it more readily.
3. Screen the patient to provide privacy.
4. Cover the patient with a bath blanket. The bath blanket is used as a drape instead of the sheet or bedspread.
5. Fill the pitcher with 250 ml or ½ pint of the solution. If tap water is used, test it with the bath thermometer.
6. Place a plastic square under the patient's hips to protect the bed. A bedpan or pad is placed over the plastic square to contain the overflow. Selection depends on the type of surgery the patient has had.
7. Ask the patient to flex the knees and keep them well apart to expose the perineal area. In proctocolectomy, the buttocks are together. A Gomco suction with irrigating apparatus is in use to remove serous drainage

and blood that occurs in the healing process (approximately 4 days). Catheters must also be considered. The patient may have one in the rectal defect and one in the bladder.

8. Pour a small amount of the solution over the inner thigh area to test its temperature against the sensitivity of the patient to the heat.
9. Hold the pitcher about 4 inches from the perineal site and pour slowly over the vulva of the female patient. Pouring avoids suture trauma or irritation and stimulates blood flow. It may be necessary to repeat this step several times in order to clear the vulva. Care must be taken to avoid contamination in the vaginal area.
10. The foreskin of the uncircumcised male patient should be retracted during the cleansing and then returned to its natural position to relieve the patient of any discomfort and avoid unnecessary swelling.
11. Use cotton balls in forceps to clean the catheter(s) of all dried blood and secretions. Forceps that are kept in disinfectant solution should be well rinsed before the procedure begins.
12. Wash the general perineal area and the legs.
13. Place clean cotton balls in the forceps and pat the area to dry. After a downward stroke toward the rectum, never reuse the cotton ball. Discarded cotton balls should be placed in a plastic bag for disposal, not dropped in the wastebasket.
14. If the patient has perineal sutures, note the condition of the sutures. Also note the presence of edema, inflammation, or any unusual drainage or excessive bleeding.
15. Apply ointment to the meatus with a sterile applicator if ordered by the physician.
16. Turn the patient to one side to check the rectal area. Hold the pitcher 4 inches from this site and pour the solution slowly over the anal area. This helps to prevent fecal contamination of the catheter and cleanse the patient.
17. Clean the rectal catheter with cotton balls held in forceps. Stroke from front to back to avoid contamination.
18. If a peri-pad is indicated, place it on the area starting from front to back.
19. Remove the plastic square and bedpan and leave the patient in a comfortable position.
20. Wash the soiled forceps with soap and water and place them in a container of disinfectant solution. This ensures clean instruments when the procedure must be repeated later in the day.
21. Discard the plastic bag with the soiled cotton balls into a covered container and return the peri-care tray to its proper place.
22. Wash hands and unscreen the patient.
23. Chart the procedure.

For irrigation of rectal defect. To control any necrosis and to clean the area, the rectal defect is irrigated every 6 or 12 hours with water or medicated solution as ordered by the physician.

1. Turn the patient to one side for ease of catheter insertion.
2. Place an ABD pad under the patient's side near the rectal area to collect the solution as it is returned.
3. Fill a 50 ml syringe with tap water or a prescription mixed in the pharmacy as ordered by the physician.
4. Insert the No. 18 catheter until it is in contact with the posterior wall (2 to 4 inches according to body structure).
5. Connect the syringe to the catheter and allow the solution to run under low gravity slowly into the catheter. The syringe should be held no higher than 4 inches above the catheter site.
6. With a cotton ball in the forceps, pat the area dry and discard the cotton ball after each stroke.
7. Remove the soiled pad and place it in a plastic bag.
8. Replace the pad as indicated.
9. Discard all soiled disposable items. Clean and return other items to the proper place.
10. Chart the procedure.

For sitz bath—chair. Sitz baths may be given twice daily unless otherwise indicated by increased drainage and discomfort.

1. Use a graduate or basin and fill the bottom of the chair about two thirds full of water 105° to 110° F. Test the water with a bath thermometer after it is in the chair.
2. Screen the patient and explain the treatment. Some hospitals have special sitz bath rooms, or the chair may be placed beside the patient's bed or in the bathroom.
3. Place a bath mat on the floor in front of the chair and a folded bath towel across the bottom of the chair where the patient's legs will touch the chair rim. Another towel over the back of the chair adds to the patient's comfort.
4. Place a glass of juice easily accessible to the patient. This action serves a twofold purpose. It replaces fluids that are so important to the ostomy patient, and the sipping of juice during the bath serves as diversional therapy.
5. Assist the patient out of bed and into the chair. Hold the chair to avoid spilling water.
6. Place the patient's bath blanket across the shoulders, down the sides, and over the knees to avoid chilling.
7. If this is the patient's first sitz bath or if conditions warrant it, stay with the patient. If the patient can be left alone, place the signal light cord within easy reach. The patient may become faint or dizzy, and the nurse should have an ampule of spirits of ammonia available at all

times. Many ostomy nurses carry these ampules in their pockets or ostomy bags.

8. Allow the patient to remain in the chair for the length of time the sitz bath is ordered. This may vary from 5 to 30 minutes, but the usual time allotment is 20 minutes. The healing therapy is more effective if the water is kept at the correct temperature. The water should be tested and warmed if the bath time is over 20 minutes. Warm water should not be added while the patient is seated. Each time the bath thermometer is used, it should be washed and sprayed with disinfectant.
9. When the bath is completed, assist the patient to stand and dry the buttocks by gently patting with the bath towel. Help the patient to bed and care for his needs.
10. Remove the seat section of the chair and empty the water into the commode or utility sink. Wash this section with soap and water and spray it with disinfectant. All items used for this procedure should be clean. The perineal area is very susceptible to infection.
11. Place all soiled linen in the hamper and chart the procedure. Charting should include treatment given, length of time, temperature of the water, and the effect of the procedure on the patient or any changes in the patient's condition.

For sitz bath—tub. The tub bath preparations and care of the patient are similar to those detailed for the sitz chair. It is important that the bathroom be free of drafts. Water in the tub should be of the same temperature as for the chair and deep enough to cover the patient's buttocks.

For portable sitz bath—pan. Portable sitz bath pans or basins are available from some surgical supply manufacturers.* These are similar to a deep wash basin, but the rims are wide enough to fit on the commode. Tubing is supplied with the set for running water into the pan.

For lamping. After the perineal area has been cleansed and the sitz bath given, the patient may be lamped to promote drying and healing.

1. Turn the patient to one side. The position of the patient will vary according to the surgery the patient has undergone. Some patients may be placed in stirrups to lamp the perineal area. If the patient cannot be turned, an attendant may hold the patient's buttocks so that heat from the lamp may be focused on the operative area.
2. Ask the patient to bring the knees forward to expose the perineal and anal area. Place a pillow under the patient's knees.
3. Place a gooseneck lamp approximately 10 inches from the perineal area.
4. Cover the exposed areas of the patient's body with towels.
5. Lamp for approximately 15 minutes.
6. Chart the procedure.

---

*One source is the Vollragh Manufacturing Co., Sheboygan, Wis.

Loop colostomy

Rinsing the loop of the intestine with warm water is soothing to the patient and will not harm the intestine. A washcloth and a pan of lukewarm water (without soap) should be used. The cloth should not be wrung out but placed dripping wet over the loop of the intestine. It should be left for a few seconds until it cools. The soiled cloth is discarded and the procedure repeated until the loop is clean. The skin is carefully patted dry with a moist cloth to remove excess water and fanned to dry.

Geriatric patient

The large intestine is one of the more common sites of disease in the elderly patient. Postoperative complications are frequent and infection is a major hazard. Because of the complexities of the older patient, good nursing care is required. The patient must be turned to prevent decubiti, and the nutritional status and electrolyte balance must be carefully watched. Because the blood circulation is poorer in this patient, he is usually colder and will require more blankets for warmth.

Infant

Care of the infant's ostomy will be decided by the physician and nurse in charge. A major concern with infants is skin excoriation. Karaya powder mixed with perianal cream and applied to the skin is a good barrier. A small appliance may be designed for the newborn ostomate by utilizing a newborn urine collector bag and the smallest size disposable nipple. The nipple, which is inserted into the urine bag opening, should be slanted with one side higher than the other in order to deflect the fecal stream. This appliance is held in place on the baby's abdomen by the adhesive backing of the urine bag and should be changed each shift. The sandwich receptacle is another approach to infant small bowel ostomy or fistula monitoring of effluent and the prevention of excoriation. This involves sandwiching a condom or Texas catheter between two disks of Reliaseal or Stomahesive and aligning the disk aperature with the stoma.

Keeping an appliance in place may become a problem when caring for an active infant. The nurse may prefer two diapers instead of a pouch. Lubricant may be added to several folded tissues and placed over the stoma before diapering the baby.

Nurses and parents will work closely together in the postoperative care of the ostomy infant. The parents must learn to care independently for the infant before he is discharged to their care.

Colostomy irrigation

The physician will decide when irrigations are to be initiated during the postoperative period. The patient is taught the irrigation procedure and may learn to assume the responsibility for performing the irrigations before he is discharged.

Temporary colostomies are seldom irrigated, since only a small segment of the bowel is available for storing fecal material and the colostomy will not regulate. An intact pouch is essential.

Most permanent colostomies are irrigated every other day. A regular commercial irrigating set should be used in the hospital so that the patient can learn the technique on the actual set he will use at home.

Equipment

Irrigating set with cone
Folded tissues
Nonsterile cotton balls
One package of Castile soap
Tincture of benzoin spray, skin prep, or skin barrier wafers
Stomahesive, Skin Bond, Stoma Reliaseal, Colly-Seels
Standard (to support the irrigating container)
Sponge rubber square, approximately 18 × 18 inches
Pitcher of liquid (juice, tea, water) for the patient to sip. Sipping liquids helps with peristalsis and alleviates nervousness in the patient.

Procedure

Preparing the irrigation bag

1. Fill the irrigation bag with 1,500 ml of tepid water and hang the bag on a standard at the patient's shoulder level. (The bottom of the bag should be no higher than shoulder level.)
2. Rid tubing of air by allowing a small portion of water to run through it.

Preparing and seating the patient

1. Face the patient's chair toward the commode and place a sponge rubber padding on the chair for the patient's comfort. (Sponge rubber is more comfortable than inflatable rubber rings.)
2. Reverse the patient's gown, but do not overexpose the patient, since chilling may occur.
3. Seat the patient comfortably and cover the knees with a bath towel. Folded tissues may be placed on the towel for convenience when needed.
4. Place a pitcher of liquid near the patient so he may sip the liquid as desired.

*Digital dilation.** A tranquilizer is helpful to combat the natural nervous apprehension of the patient and should be given 30 minutes before the dilating procedure begins.

1. Explain the procedure to alleviate the patient's fear of his stoma.
2. Teach him the direction of the colon.

---

*This procedure may not always be necessary.

3. Place a rubber examining glove on the patient's hand and lubricate the forefinger with stoma lubricant. (Many patients use the small finger.)
4. Place folded tissues under the stoma to contain any mucus or fecal matter that might be expelled.
5. Take the patient's hand and guide his finger into the stoma, gently but firmly, for at least 2 inches. Hold his finger in the stoma for 1 minute to dilate the stoma.
6. If bright red blood is noted when the patient removes his finger, reassure the patient that this will happen occasionally. Mucosa bleeds readily but there is no danger of hemorrhage.

Placing the irrigating sleeve

1. Apply stoma lubricant to the stoma.
2. Moisten the gasket on the irrigating sleeve with water to prevent backflow.
3. Place the irrigating sleeve on the patient and fasten the belt.

Inserting the cone

1. Insert the irrigating cone, allowing water to run slowly.
2. Open the tubing to allow inflow.
3. Ask the patient to breathe deeply while the irrigant is entering the colon. *Never force* the cone; always remove it, relax, and try again. If insertion is unsuccessful after several attempts, notify the physician.
4. When the irrigation is completed, remove the cone and let the patient rest for 15 minutes in order the allow the first backflow.
5. Fold the bottom of the irrigating sleeve twice, clipping the fold to the top of the sleeve to make a temporary catch bag.
6. If the patient is ambulatory, help him robe and instruct him to walk 10 minutes. (Movement is desirable for good elimination.)
7. In approximately 30 minutes return the patient to the bathroom and seat him on a chair.
8. To rinse the sleeve, fill the temporary bag with water and let it run through the sleeve.
9. Remove the sleeve and wipe the colostomy with tissues. Wash the stoma and surrounding area with mild soap and water. Rinse and dry thoroughly.
10. Cover the stoma with a cotton ball and spray the surrounding area with tincture of benzoin.
11. Apply the stoma pouch.

Irrigation notes

1. A solution of a 1-ounce package of Castile soap to 1 quart of water may prove successful if irrigations are slow to return.
2. If cramps occur during irrigation, the water may be too cold or the flow of water into the tube may be too rapid.
3. Regularity is obtained by irrigating at the same time of day.

4. The permanent colostomy will require approximately 6 weeks to regulate through use of diet and irrigation. Until then, a cemented-on disposable stoma pouch should be used for protection and peace of mind.
5. After regulation has been achieved, the pouch may be eliminated. Several thicknesses of tissues with petrolatum on one side may be placed over the stoma. A square of plastic wrap placed on top of these tissues will prevent moisture from seeping through. This dressing may be held in place with a wide elastic band or a stretch girdle.
6. When the patient becomes confident and learns control, he rarely wears an appliance between irrigations except for protection when traveling or for a long day when it may be inconvenient to irrigate.

As the patient progresses from acute care to convalescent care, the nurse-patient relationship should be constructive, not dependent. When the patient is discharged from the hospital, he should be confident in the ''how to'' of ostomy self-care.

Contraindications to irrigation

1. Irritable bowel syndrome
2. Ascending or transverse colostomies
3. Mentally retarded patient
4. Arthritic joints

COMPLICATIONS COMMON TO COLONIC OPERATIONS*

1. Sepsis
2. Ileus
3. Hemorrhage
4. Fistula
5. Pulmonary emboli
6. Thrombi
7. Dehiscence and evisceration
8. Urinary tract infections
9. Cardiovascular accidents
10. Cerebrovascular accidents
11. Peritonitis
12. Abscess

Factors that increase incidence

1. Age and physiologic condition
2. Ulcerative colitis
3. Malnutrition and electrolyte imbalance
4. Obstruction
5. Bleeding
6. Anemia

---

*Contributed by Christine Mahar, LPNET Tucson Medical Center.

7. Collateral circulation trauma
8. Anastomotic leaks
9. Length of operative procedure and time anesthetized

Methods to prevent complications

1. Correlation of diagnostic facts
2. Mechanical bowel preparation
3. Nasogastric tube
4. Foley catheter
5. Changing position, deep breathing, coughing
6. Use of antibiotics
7. Oral elemental diet
8. Early ambulation

Complications of transverse colostomy

1. Wound abscess
2. Herniation
3. Retraction, prolapse

Complications of sigmoid colostomy

1. Stricture at skin level
2. Hemorrhage
3. Hernia
4. Retraction, prolapse

Complications of ileostomy

1. Electrolyte imbalance
2. Ileus
3. Stricture, prolapse
4. Fistula
5. Hernia
6. Dermatitis circumostomy

CHAPTER 8

Care of the dying patient

Death is understandably a stress subject; the fact that all life ends is often difficult to accept. This cannot always be counted as a negative experience, however, for death is a biological part of life and sometimes the solution to life's insurmountable problems. Each dying patient's situation must be evaluated and a close doctor-nurse liaison formed in order to establish a nursing plan suitable to that individual.

Knowing that a patient is dying is an emotional experience for the staff. Since the dying process exists and cannot be halted for a particular patient, a feeling of helplessness is created in all those who attend him. Staff members often experience stress because of the inability to talk freely to the patient, and they are uncomfortable in his company. The game of false pretense sometimes played by the family and patient adds to the tension of the situation.

In ostomy surgery, as in every other field of surgery, some patients will die in spite of all that medical science can offer. The dying ostomy patient, because of his special circumstances, requires more supportive understanding and personal attention than other patients. For this patient the initial stage of dying begins even before surgery, and the process may encompass many hospital admissions and releases before death finally occurs. This is an especially traumatic experience for the family and patient; both will require much counseling and support from staff members who are in attendance during this period. A program of care should be established based on the particular physical and emotional needs of the patient.

It is the physician who determines what information regarding the patient's illness and approaching death the patient or family receives, but a general procedure of supportive care is the responsibility of the staff in both plan and performance.

MEETING PHYSICAL AND EMOTIONAL NEEDS OF THE DYING PATIENT

Program of physical care

Pain and discomfort. The patient should be kept comfortable by the use of medications. His comfort may be increased by the aid of pillows or sheepskin

☐ Contributed by Lillian Frye, R.N., Nursing Supervisor, Tucson Medical Center.

placed under pressure areas and frequent adjustment of the body position. As body positions are changed, massage will promote a relaxed attitude. Passive exercises such as arm movements and use of pedals for the legs will alleviate muscle strain. Body temperature may be controlled. If the patient is cold, socks may be placed on his feet and more blankets may be added for warmth. Cool drinks, a room temperature below 70°, and washing the patient's face with cool water will be refreshing to the patient who is too warm.

Odor. A nursing staff with a positive attitude will involve the patient in conversation to divert his attention from worry about odor. Feelings of disgust about the malodor in the room must not be communicated to the patient. Cleanliness and the use of deodorizers are essential to odor control; therefore the pouch should be cleaned of fecal drainage one or two times each 8-hour shift, and deodorant should be placed in the pouch after it is cleaned. Spraying the body and the bed linen with deodorants and keeping the general room surroundings fresh and clean will promote a more acceptable atmosphere.

Program of emotional care

Patient's emotional needs. An alert nursing staff can perceive the patient's feelings of desertion and confusion and show concern. Members of the staff who are preoccupied with their own feelings will fail to recognize the patient's unconscious awareness of approaching death. The manner of the nurses' initial response to the patient's needs often influences his ability to adjust to the situation.

Each day, if possible, the same personnel should care for the patient to promote a feeling of security. A relaxed atmosphere, a personal touch, sharing a cup of tea or coffee with the patient, or taking him out of the room at intervals will demonstrate to the patient that he is special.

The patient needs to feel free to express his hope of eventual recovery or even his negative feelings toward himself and his situation. Considerate nurses who deal with the patient's questions will ask for more information and reflect back the patient's opinion, not their own. If the patient requests religious counseling, the nurse should secure this help for him.

As the disease progresses, the patient will enter stages of anger, resentment, depression, and finally the acceptance of death. His anger and resentment of the fact that he is dying are often directed toward the nurse through verbal tirade. Instead of becoming resentful, the nurse should remain objective, allow the patient to relieve his feelings, and consistently continue visits to the patient's room regardless of his negative response.

Depressive behavior takes the form of moodiness and unresponsiveness on the part of the patient. It is, in effect, the patient mourning his own death. Little attentions will help lift this depression. The patient should have a bed near the window of a quiet room on the unit—not isolated but less confused.

Diversional therapy will often break the monotony of the patient's long day and result in pleasant memories. If the patient is able to leave his room, he may be taken to visit other patients, lunch on the patio, or attend a movie.

Some patients find it difficult to accept the fact of death while others are able, in the final stage, to slowly and peacefully detach themselves and accept it. The nurse should continue frequent visits to the patient's bedside and encourage the family to support the patient with their presence.

No amount of planning, care, and support can totally ease the emotional and physical pain experienced by the terminally ill patient. This patient must come to terms not only with pain but also with death, in his own fashion. A program of care for the patient that frees him from unnecessary pain and stress will increase his ability to cope with his own situation.

Family's emotional need. Involving the family in the patient's care will ease their feelings of helplessness by providing them with something to do. They can help with the daily bath and bed change, feed the patient, and assist in stoma care. Close association of the family with the patient should be encouraged to reassure the patient that he is not repugnant and to satisfy the family's desire to feel needed.

CHAPTER 9

Skin care

The skin, an important organ of the body, is made up of sweat and oil glands, nerve fibers, and thousands of cells. The epidermis is the outer surface of the skin, the protective sheath, described as stratified squamous epithelium. The underlying layer, the dermis, reproduces new cells that multiply and move to the surface. The dead cells shed and are replaced by these new cells. The epidermis has no blood vessels, but the deeper layers of the skin have fine nerve fibers that serve as sensors to indicate discomfort.

Decreased circulation and the degeneration of cells in aging affects the skin; it becomes drier and thinner and heals more slowly.

The ostomy patient has a particular need for well-maintained skin because of the additional wear and tear to which his skin will be subjected. Emphasis must therefore be placed on the health of skin around any stoma or orifice. The skin varies in thickness on different parts of the body, being thickest where it is most exposed to friction and thinnest on the anterior surface of the trunk where stomas are placed. Each individual's skin reacts differently to medications and treatments, and it is capable of rejecting a treatment that has been successful in other cases.

The nightmare of the ostomy patient is skin excoriation. The word ''excoriation'' is derived from *ex,* out, and *corium,* skin, meaning an abrasion or scratching of the epidermis. Skin excoriation refers to the irritated skin surrounding the stoma or fistula.

The patient with an ileostomy has a greater problem from effluent than the colostomy patient does. The ileostomy stool is liquid and contains digestive enzymes. The stool from the colostomy is soft to formed in consistency, depending on which segment of the colon is surgically involved. If the skin is not protected from the enzymes or if the appliance is undermined, the effluent will come in contact with the outer layer of the skin, causing excoriation.

Skin problems can be kept to a minimum if the staff is aware of the necessity of maintaining the integrity of the skin circumostomy. Proper fitting of the temporary appliance and preparation of the skin at the outset will eliminate most of these problems.

Fecal effluent may contact any area of the body. Many surgeons prevent skin damage from effluent by applying a temporary pouch after surgery instead of dressings that allow drainage to seep through and touch unprotected skin. In the recovery room the pouch or dressings should be checked for signs of leakage and skin irritation.

There are many types of skin excoriation, and each type requires a different skin care procedure.

The best cleansing agent for the skin is nondetergent soap and water.

Normal skin

1. Loosen the adhesive on the body with a solvent and carefully remove the appliance one corner at a time to prevent skin tearing around the stoma.
2. Place a stoma drain or wick over the stoma and an emesis basin under the drain. The flow from the stoma is directed away from the skin into the basin while the stoma is being cleaned. The stoma empties out at any time, and the effluent must be contained to prevent damage to the skin.
3. If a stoma drain is not available, use a 1-inch wide Penrose drain or a deflector fashioned from a 3-inch piece of Telfa surgical dressing, rolled to cylinder size of the stoma. Place cotton balls over the stoma if the drainage is slight.
4. Wash the skin with warm water and soap. The soap in the patient's room may be used unless the patient is allergic to it. Carefully avoid contact with the stoma for the first week, since a new stoma is delicate and bleeds easily.
5. Rinse well. Make certain that all soap is removed from the skin so that the adhesive will adhere.
6. Fan to dry or use the cool setting on an electric hair dryer.
7. Cover the stoma and spray circumostomy with tincture of benzoin following the physician's order. Hold the spray can 4 inches from the skin for a smooth spray.
8. Apply the clean appliance. (See Chapter 10.)

Change in color of skin. The skin may assume different shades of blue, red, or purple. This may occur following surgery or may result from a diminished blood supply or belt pressure. Skin that has come in contact with stoma drainage and has been slightly burned may be bright red, like diaper rash. If discoloration is found after the pouch is removed, try the following:

1. Place the stoma drain or a deflector over the stoma.
2. Cleanse the skin with warm water and soap.
3. Rinse well and dry.
4. Spray with tincture of benzoin to toughen the skin.
5. To ease the pressure of the pouch against the stoma, use one of several available products such as Reliaseal, Stomahesive, or karaya seals.
6. Apply a thin layer of surgical cement around the stoma to increase wearability of the pouch.
7. Dry thoroughly. The cement must be dry or the pad will not success-

fully adhere. A double-faced Stomaseal may be used instead of surgical cement and does not require drying time.
8. Place the skin barrier snugly around the stoma.
9. Cover the top of the skin barrier with surgical cement.
10. Apply the pouch. (See Chapter 10.)

Weeping skin. Skin left untreated after coming in contact with effluent becomes burned as the skin is digested. If further neglected, the skin will become excoriated and weepy. For this problem the following steps may be taken:

1. Remove the appliance with Detachol or other noncaustic solvent. Do not use caustic solvents on irritated skin.
2. Place a drain or wick over the stoma.
3. Wash the skin well with soap and water.
4. Rinse and dry well.
5. Use a gooseneck lamp with a 60-watt bulb to dry the skin and encourage healing. Hold the lamp 6 to 8 inches away from the stoma area for approximately 8 minutes. Do *not* use a sunlamp.
6. Spray with tincture of benzoin unless the excoriation is too extensive.
7. Using a cotton ball on the pad of the finger, apply an aluminum hydroxide compound such as Amphojel to the area.
8. Let the application dry for 2 or 3 minutes to a chalky white.
9. Spray karaya powder on the white area. Dust it with a cotton ball toward the stoma, to absorb the moisture of weeping.
10. Let the powder dry to a hard crust, forming a strong base for the surgical cement.
11. Dust away any particles of loose powder.
12. Apply surgical cement thinly. Cover the powdered area well.
13. Allow to dry thoroughly.
14. Apply the pouch. (See Chapter 10.)

Through this process, a new thickness between the patient's skin and the pouch has been created. If the pouch is undermined during the next 24 hours, the skin layer will not be damaged further.

Sloughing. Sloughing is the formation of dead tissue that has been cast out of or is still contained in living tissue. Pressure of the faceplate or the appliance belt or an infection can cause sloughing to occur circumostomy. This is a condition that must be evaluated by the surgeon or ostomy nurse. There are several methods of caring for sloughing.

Aluminum hydroxide gel (Amphojel) and karaya powder should be applied to the skin in layers until a thick gummy protective coating is built up. The appliance will adequately adhere to this mixture without cement. When it is necessary to replace the mixture, *only* that which is deeply soiled is cleaned off and more karaya and Amphojel applied. Badly excoriated skin will heal rapidly under such a coating if given the opportunity.

If sloughing continues, the appliance is removed and the patient placed face down on a Stryker frame, allowing the stoma to drain into a receptacle. The Stryker frame treatment may be used until the patient's skin has had time to air. During this period, the skin is treated with antisepetics and steroid sprays.

In extreme cases plastic surgery may be performed.

Other problems

Subskin orifice caused by pancreatic fistula. It is very difficult to control and prevent skin excoriation from this extremely caustic drainage. A sump pump may be used if ordered by the physician.

Resting the skin. The pouch should not be removed from the stoma or ointments and dressings applied in an attempt to rest the skin. This procedure will further complicate the situation. Dressings retain the moist effluents and allow them to spread to other parts of the body. The drain and an emesis basin may be used for several hours to allow the skin to rest. If convenient, a Stryker frame may be used.

Allergy to skin cement. Allergy is most often a result of a particular solvent in the cement. A brand that uses another type of solvent should be substituted or the stoma pouch applied without cement. If the problem persists, a non-allergenic, pressure-sensitive, silicone spray adhesive should be used around the stoma.

Skin irritation caused by yeast invasion. Skin irritation under the disk caused by yeast invasion will respond to nystatin (Mycostatin) or a steroid powder. A very small amount is sprinkled on clean skin and dusted in well; then the appliance is applied as usual. If no yeast is visible but the skin irritation indicates probable yeast invasion, triamcinolone (Kenalog) spray should be used. The combination of Kenalog spray and Mycostatin powder usually remedies persistent cases.

Encrustation. Sometimes skin folds around the ileal conduit stoma will collect urea crystals. If this occurs, ½ cup of white vinegar should be mixed with 1 quart of water. The mixture is placed in the bottom of the pouch twice daily (morning and bedtime). The pouch is closed, and the patient should lie down for 20 minutes to allow the solution to bathe the affected area. With a physician's advice, a silver nitrate stick may be used to remove encrustration, but it may cause bleeding.

Exanthemas. Exanthemas may occur as a result of radiotherapy treatment; this can be a toxic effect resulting from products of destroyed cancer cells or an allergic reaction. They may also occur as a result of hypersensitiveness of the patient, or be pharmacogenetically induced (refers to the study of hereditary response to drugs).

A dermatologist should be consulted to diagnose and prescribe for the patient. Frequently, systemic treatment is required instead of local antimicrobial therapy.

CHAPTER 10

Appliances

Today, appliance manufacturers are constantly researching ostomy equipment to meet a variety of needs, but the first appliances, like the first ostomy surgeries, resulted from desperation. The first colostomy bag is thought to have been a small leather bag, designed by Daguesceau in 1795, for a patient on whom he had performed a sigmoid colon surgery. Many appliances developed as a result of the experimentation of ingenious patients who sought convenient methods and comfortable appliances. A truss fitted with a tin box to catch feces was discarded in favor of a piece of soft sponge held in place with bandages, thus allowing gas to pass but retaining the feces. Resourceful patients used whatever means were available to allow them to return to normal activities, while other patients went into retirement until the day they died.

An ''appliance,'' according to medical dictionaries, is a device affixed to or implanted in the body and designed to take the place of or perform the function of a missing body part. To some ostomy patients, ''appliance'' is an important word because the patient is exchanging a part of the body for a functional device. If the nursing staff is oriented to the proper use of appliances, the patient is assured of an established routine. Thorough instruction in ostomy management builds the patient's confidence in his own abilities and promotes favorable adjustment to his new life.

The designated ostomy surgery dictates whether an appliance is necessary. In some cases catheters, tracheal tubes, or dressings are utilized.

There are two classes of appliances: permanent and temporary. Temporary appliances are disposable pouches, used postoperatively until the stoma has sufficiently healed and a permanent appliance has been selected. In general, permanent appliances are those which can be cleaned and reused. A permanent faceplate may accommodate either a temporary or a permanent pouch. Use of the permanent appliance is not feasible or recommended until approximately 6 weeks after surgery, or until edema disappears and the stoma matures.

Appliance manufacturers include basic instructions with each product. The ostomate learns to adapt these instructions to his own body by experimenting to determine the adaptability of the product to his various needs; for example, wearing the appliance in the bathtub before going swimming. Proper adjustment to the appliance is evidenced by the unlimited sports activities in which ostomates participate.

GUIDELINES IN SELECTING OSTOMY APPLIANCES AND ACCESSORIES

Appliances are manufactured in various sizes to accommodate anatomic variances of patients—newborn, pediatric, regular, and extra large sizes.

As with foods, choosing the proper appliance is a trial and error process until the ostomy patient discovers the one that best meets individual needs. An appliance may be purchased in a set, or parts of the appliance may be obtained from different manufacturers and assembled to satisfy individual requirements. The ostomy nurse, who is experienced in the foibles of appliances, is an excellent resource for information in the selection of the appropriate appliance. Buying in small quantities until there has been time for experimentation is wise.

Selecting stoma size opening. An ideal stoma size is 1 inch in diameter with a projecting spout of 1 inch. The spout is necessary to ensure that all drainage goes into the appliance and does not come into contact with the skin. Each stoma is individual in size and shape and the aperture of the appliance or faceplate must be carefully measured. An opening that is too large will allow leakage to occur, and one that is too small will result in constriction of the stoma. Care should be taken to ensure that a $^{1}/_{8}$- to $^{1}/_{16}$-inch space is maintained between the appliance and the stoma. A stoma-measuring guide may be used to align the center orifice of the faceplate with the stoma.

Faceplates. The faceplate should be very carefully selected, with special consideration given to wearability. Full body movement and normal physical activities are facilitated by the use of flexible or light-weight plastic body rings, worn with or without a belt. Some plates are malleable and easily adjusted to fit the contour of the abdominal wall surrounding the stoma, thereby ensuring a tight, leakproof seal. Smooth beveled edges around the aperture of the faceplate will prevent the edges from cutting into the stoma. Permanent faceplates should be removed weekly or as often as indicated by discomfort or leakage, and the skin cleansed.

Customized faceplate. In the event that the stoma is not round, the faceplate aperture may be modified to achieve a more accurate fit. A pattern of the outer perimeter of the stoma may be sent to the manufacturer or to the hospital artisan for modification of the faceplate aperture. Many ostomy nurses have mastered the art of customizing faceplates, thus providing immediate service to the patient.

Artisans of Tucson Medical Center provide a complimentary custom fit to their ostomy patients. The ostomy nurse transfers the patient's pattern to the faceplates before sending them for customizing. The artisan sets a wooden dowel in a vise and secures the faceplate on the dowel.

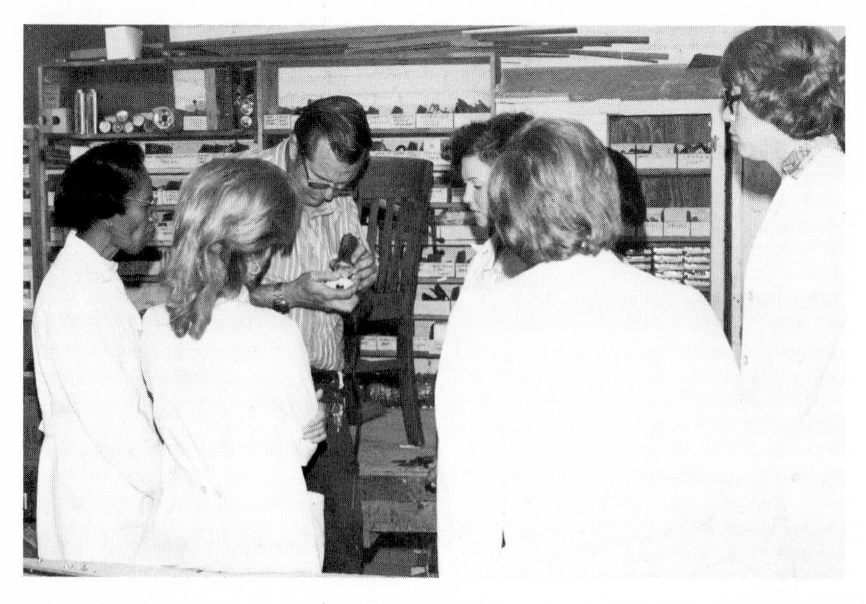

Fig. 10-1. Pete Brolund, Tucson Medical Center artisan, instructs ostomy nurse students in the art of faceplate customizing.

White soft faceplates are cut with a No. 11 surgical blade to the approximate size as marked. The knife is inserted into the pattern line and held steady while the faceplate is rotated around the knife blade to avoid irregular cutting. A cone stone, attached to the Dremel Moto Tool, is used to bevel the opening.

Gray hard rubber faceplates with convexity cannot be cut with the surgical blade. A $^{3}/_{16}$-inch router bit is used to cut the opening to an approximate size, and beveling is accomplished to round out the opening.

Belts. Ostomates may or may not wear a belt except for security reasons at night or when traveling. Belts come with various connecting adjustments, buckles, and hooks. The weight, composition, and width are personal preferences and can be modified to individual needs.

A retainer is fastened around the faceplate and the belt is connected to the retainer. A loose belt may cause the appliance to pull away from the skin; an overtight belt may cause skin problems or ulcers. Neoprene rubber belts may be worn for swimming or whenever a tight belt is required. Spraying the belts with Scotchgard will waterproof them to a certain degree, and powder under the belt will help to prevent chafing.

Pouches. Temporary pouches are usually applied in surgery. These disposable pouches with adhesive backings are available in all sizes to accommodate drainage of surgical wounds and ostomies. Pouches are manufac-

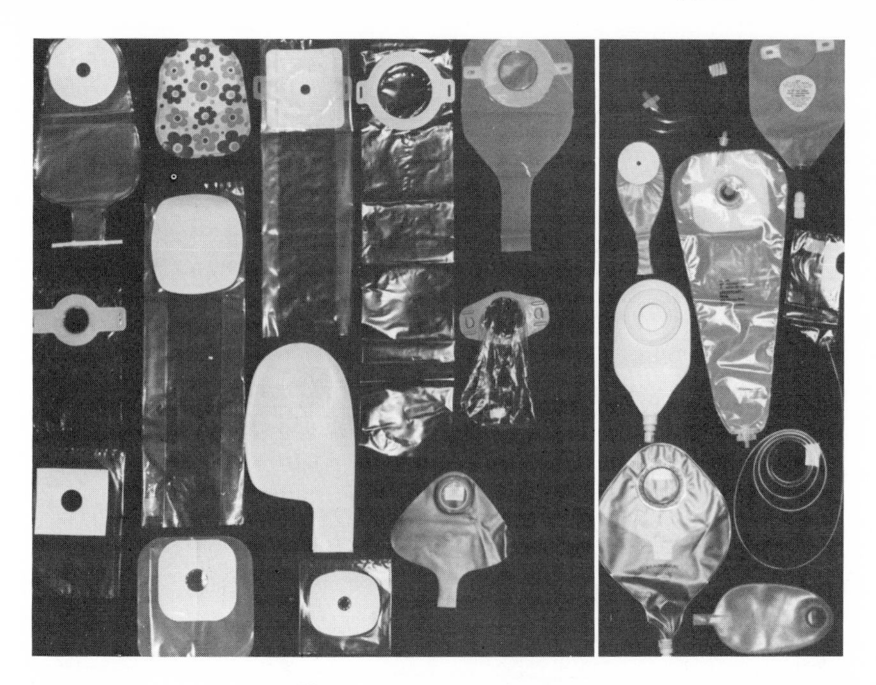

Fig. 10-2. Collection pouches.

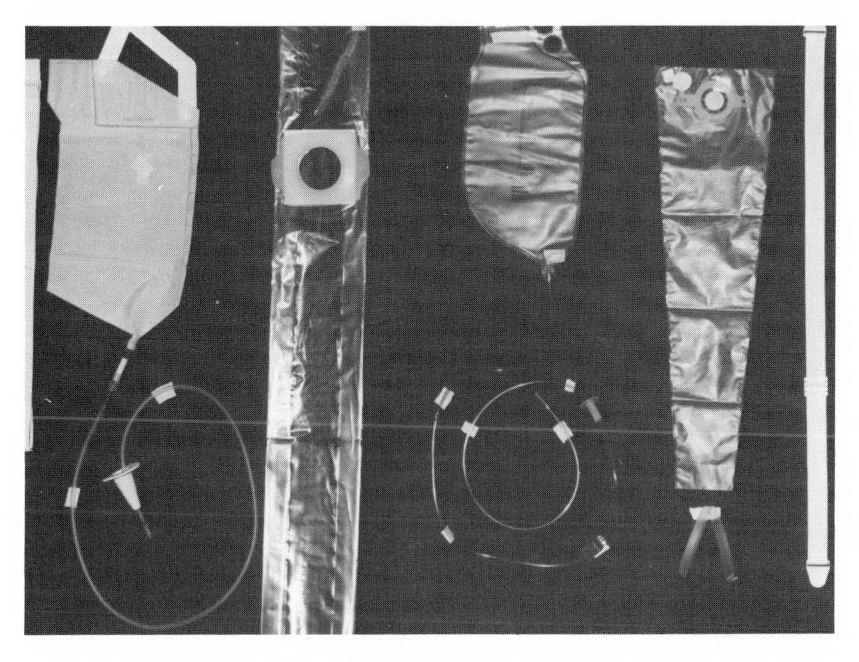

Fig. 10-3. Irrigating appliances and sleeves.

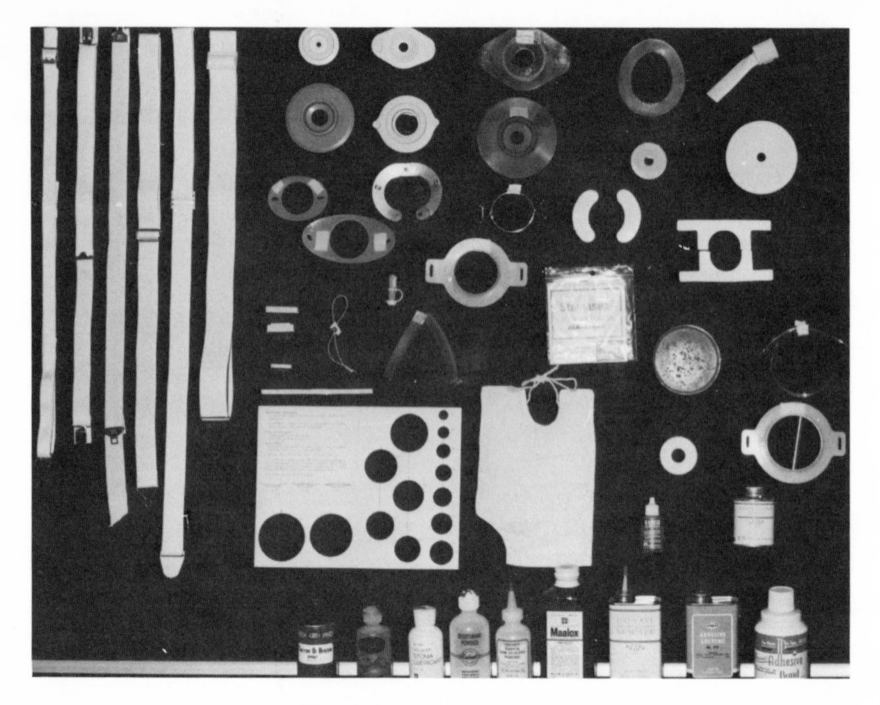

Fig. 10-4. Ostomy accessories.

tured from combinations of various rubber and synthetic materials. A one-piece appliance is available for those who require this convenience.

Urine collection pouches are usually made of latex or lightweight vinyl. Fecal stream diversion requires an odor-preventing pouch, either vinyl or synthetic rubber, although many patients prefer to use disposable plastic pouches for this purpose.

Each patient must evaluate the pouch as to weight, size, comfort, and ease of emptying without upsetting normal dressing habits.

Ostomy accessories. Many accessories are manufactured by ostomy supply companies. A few of the most common accessories are as follows:

1. Stomahesive, Reliaseal, and karaya disks are used as gaskets.
2. Finger cots may be used for stoma dilation in lieu of rubber gloves.
3. Karaya gum powder or paste, used as a protective base, allows the skin to heal. Appliances adhere easily to this base.
4. Instead of mixing the karaya gum powder to form a karaya worm, a karaya gum washer may be moistened and then stretched or cut to fit snugly around the stoma.
5. Very thin, double-faced adhesive disks will adhere to the faceplate, appliance, or skin and are often used instead of cement.

6. Cements and adhesives are available in a tube or a can with an applicator.
7. Solvents may be used to dissolve cement and adhesives and are necessary for removing the appliance. A noncaustic oil base solvent is available for those with tender skin (Detachol).
8. Telfa is a sterile, nonadhering dressing that allows excoriated skin to heal without further damage.
9. Micropore, a paper tape, is a nonallergenic tape for those who are unable to use adhesive tape.
10. Stoma bibs made of diaper cloth or cotton flannel fit under the plastic pouch to absorb perspiration and keep the appliance from contacting the skin.
11. O'Rings, made of covered elastic thread, may be stretched slightly to fit around the disk to secure the pouch.
12. Rubber rings or plastic valve sets may be utilized as pouch closures.
13. Plastic drying hangers hold the pouch open for airing.
14. Colostomy shields may be worn over the stoma after irrigation for protection.
15. Night hook-up tubing for gravity drainage is available in various lengths and adaptors for urinary diversion.

PRIMARY UTILIZATION OF APPLIANCES

Patient in surgery. Instead of using dressings over the stoma, many surgeons prefer to apply temporary pouches for skin protection. If the first outpourings are collected in a pouch, the physician may examine the effluent and, at the same time, protect the patient's skin from contact with enzymatic drainage. When a pouch is applied in surgery, the skin area around the stoma should be cleansed of natural oils by using an alcohol swab to facilitate adherence of the pouch.

Patient in recovery room. Dressings or pouches are seldom changed in the recovery room, since gut activity normally does not resume for 12 hours; however, they are checked.

Patient in his room. The temporary pouch is usually not removed for 3 days, which enables the physician to watch for possible edema and to observe the stoma. The stoma pouch should be checked daily for signs of undermining. Should leakage occur, a new pouch must be applied promptly. A stoma at skin level will require more observation to maintain an intact seal.

CHANGING AND REPLACING THE APPLIANCE

Checking the ostomy site and gathering supplies. The ostomy site should be checked for activity. If the appliance is changed before the patient eats, there will be less effluent during the change. All necessary supplies should be gathered and placed on a table, ready for immediate use.

Removing faceplate or adhesive disk. The disk or faceplate should not be removed more often than necessary, since too frequent change may injure the skin before it is desensitized to tapes, seals, and cements. Initially, the faceplate may be removed every other day unless leakage necessitates prior removal. As experience develops, the patient may wear a disk or plate for many days or as long as the skin remains in good condition. An especially well-fitting disk or plate may be worn as long as a month.

A nonallergenic solvent should always be used to loosen the faceplate or disk. Starting at one edge, the patient moistens the adhesive with a cotton ball saturated in solvent or uses a medicine dropper of solvent, a drop at a time, as the disk or plate is slowly removed. The faceplate or disk should not be pulled off with one movement.

The faceplate is cleaned and a thin coat of adhesive spread for drying while the skin is being prepared. The skin must always be cleansed, rinsed, and dried each time an appliance is removed.

Replacing the appliance. If a specially prepared adhesive disk is not used, a thin coat of cement should be applied to the skin and allowed to become tacky. The patient may hold a mirror for better observation of the procedure.

The faceplate center is positioned over the stoma, allowing a clearance of $^1/_8$ to $^1/_{16}$ inch. A stoma shield (strip of paper coiled to fit the faceplate opening) may be placed over the stoma for more accurate placement of the plate and then removed after the plate has been pressed onto the abdomen. The faceplate is pressed into position. To avoid skin wrinkles, which could loosen the appliance, the patient should stretch the abdomen before the application.

The retainer and belt are applied. A belt is not absolutely essential in wearing a pouch but adds to security. The belt should not bind but should be snug enough to keep the pouch from moving. Proper snugness of the belt is assured when two fingers may be passed between the skin and the belt with ease.

Attaching the appliance

Fistula. A paper pattern is cut to fit around the opening of the fistula and the pattern traced on the adhesive disk of a large disposable pouch. The opening is cut to fit the pattern. The area around the fistula should be cleansed and the pouch applied over the fistula opening, the bag placed in the direction of easiest emptying. Extra strips of nonallergenic tape may be necessary to secure the pouch.

Wound dehiscence. For extensive wound dehiscence, a large plastic bag may be utilized. An opening may be cut in the bag by using a pattern of the wound area. The opening is reinforced with adhesive tape and the pouch attached to the skin with cement or tape.

Gastric drainage. Disposable stoma pouches may be utilized for gastric drainage. Improvisation of materials will be necessary in most cases, depending on the area needing protection.

To prevent leakage around drains or tubing, the tubing may be disconnected, threaded through a disposable pouch, reconnected, and the pouch cemented to the skin. Fluid accumulated in the pouch may be emptied.

Changing the ileostomy temporary appliance

1. Estimate the size of the stoma before ordering supplies. Assemble the supplies on a table near the patient.
2. Make a paper pattern of the stoma and cut an opening in the temporary pouch.
3. Secure a small plastic bag near the patient to hold soiled cotton balls or tissues.
4. Place cotton balls over the stoma to collect drainage.
5. Cleanse the skin surrounding the stoma (Chapter 9).
6. If there is an excessive amount of adhesive build-up on the skin, remove it with solvent. A small build-up will not interfere with the Stomaseal or other gaskets of choice.
7. Remove the paper backing from the stoma pouch. Apply a thin coat of cement to the adhesive surface and set aside to dry.
8. Spray the skin surrounding the stoma with tincture of benzoin or skin prep and air dry.
9. Apply a thin coat of cement close to the stoma and extend it beyond the edges where the pouch will cover. Fan to dry.
10. Apply the pouch carefully to avoid skin wrinkles.
11. Expel all air from the pouch.
12. Close the pouch by turning it up two times from the bottom and fan folding. Secure it with a rubber band or a tail closure.
13. Tape the top, bottom, and sides of the pouch with nonallergenic paper tape for added protection.

Changing the ileal conduit appliance

1. Assemble supplies on the patient's bedside stand.
2. If the patient can bend in the direction of the drain, the conduit will empty most of the urine before the appliance is changed.
3. Remove the appliance slowly with solvent to avoid excoriation of the skin.
4. Place a stoma drain over the stoma or a pill bottle with a cotton ball inside to absorb drainage.
5. Cleanse the area around the stoma and dry thoroughly.
6. Spread cement evenly on the disk and let it dry thoroughly.
7. Center the disk over the stoma and attach the belt.
8. Position the pouch so that the spout falls on the inside of the thigh. Stretch the pouch opening to fit over the flange of the disk.
9. Place nonallergenic tape around the edges of the disk to hold it in place.
10. At night, open the valve on the bottom of the pouch and attach a tube

to a container, allowing the pouch to empty. Keep the tube straight, since stagnant urine breeds bacteria. A closed-system drainage set, glass jars, or plastic bleach bottles may be used as containers.

11. Rinse the tubing and pouch daily with diluted vinegar to prevent crystal build-up, taking care not to disturb the disk. Wash the inside of the pouch with a syringe or a portable shower head spray. Rinse the pouch well and hang to dry. When dry, powder the pouch inside and out to prevent the sides from sticking together.
12. Have the patient drink cranberry juice daily to deodorize and possibly clear the urine.

Loop or double-barrel colostomy appliance. The patient with a loop or double-barrel colostomy is a challenge to the nursing staff, since the large intestinal loop or the division of the loop that creates the double-barrel colostomy will often be difficult to enclose in one pouch. This colostomy will begin to drain feces as peristalsis returns, and the drainage must be contained either by dressings or by a collection pouch.

The main concern in fitting the pouch over the loop colostomy is enclosing the rod, tube, and colostomy. Larger pouches (4- to 5-inch openings) may be used to accommodate the large loop. Some surgeons use the Marsan Loop-Loc appliance or the Hollister Loop Ostomy Bridge assembly at the time of surgery.

Pouch attachment

Procedure. The pouch opening is trimmed to fit around the stoma. A towel may be placed on a plastic square close to the patient's colostomy to prevent soiling and the skin prepared. (See Chapter 9.)

Applying the pouch. The pouch is changed as often as indicated (when the seal is broken and leaks occur) to keep the patient dry and without odor. If properly placed, the drainable pouch, emptied every 2 hours to relieve the weight and heat that collects, may remain in place for 3 to 4 days.

An assistant is a valuable asset in placing this pouch because of the large area to be covered.

The protective covering should be carefully removed from the adhesive backing. For a smoother application of the adhesive backing and to prevent wrinkles or air bubbles, the protective covering may be removed, cut into sections, replaced on the adhesive backing, and a section at a time removed as the adhesive is placed on the skin.

One hand is placed inside the pouch and the opening centered over the stoma. As the assistant holds one side of the pouch, one section of the adhesive protective covering is removed and that section firmly applied to the skin around the patient's stoma. Sections of the cover continue to be removed and pressed around the stoma until the entire disk is in place. The disk may be pressed around the stoma without sectioning the cover by starting inside and pressing out to the edge, but sectioning makes a smoother application.

Drops of deodorant are placed in the pouch and all air left in the pouch is expelled. The bottom of the pouch is folded up, fan folded, and secured with a rubber band or tail closure. The pouch is placed horizontally if the patient is bedfast and vertically if the patient is ambulatory.

The pouch should be emptied before meals and at hours of sleep for patient comfort. Regular emptying also promotes accurate output records.

CHAPTER 11

Importance of fluids and electrolytes

Approximately 3 quarts of liquid are required by the body to perform its daily function of eliminating body heat through perspiration and the excretion of body waste by means of the kidneys. Fluid requirements differ with the individual depending on age, height, weight, and body activity.

Electrolytes in the body maintain the acid-base balance and control water volume. The normal body requirements of sodium and potassium are usually met by the regular intake of nourishment.

As long as the regular routine of intake and output of water and chemicals is balanced, the body function is normal. However, when the body is under stress, body fluids are rapidly depleted through vomiting, diarrhea, and fever and must be replaced for the body to regain electrolyte balance.

Fluids are particularly important to the ostomate because dehydration can readily occur. Some ostomates are salt losers and others water losers; this will depend on how much of the colon, which absorbs most of the fluids, has been removed.

Variations of fluid intake and output should be especially observed in summer when fluids are excreted from the body at a faster rate. Ostomates who live in desert areas should be particularly cautious. The ileostomy salt output is usually 1 teaspoon a day, and extra fluids should be added to the regular diet. If there is no salt restriction for the ileostomate, extra salt may be used on foods.

Gastroenteritis (intestinal flu) associated with fever, nausea, vomiting, and diarrhea usually lasts 24 to 48 hours and is accompanied by dehydration. Gastrointestinal upsets are especially serious to the ileostomy patient. When the colon is removed, there is diminished water absorption.

The nurse should be cognizant of excessive fluid loss and inform the physician so that replacement may be initiated.

Symptoms of dehydration

1. Dry and warm skin
2. Marked thirst
3. Abdominal cramps

4. Scanty urine output
5. Shortness of breath
6. Lassitude

Replacement of fluids. If drainage is more than 1,000 ml in 24 hours, supplementary intake should be initiated. Some suggestions:

1. One 8-ounce glass of any of the following:
   Water with ½ teaspoon salt
   Water with ½ teaspoon bicarbonate of soda
   Orange juice, tomato juice, or fruit nectar
   Tea, cola, or bouillon
2. Intravenous fluids if indicated

Replacement of sodium. Sodium is necessary to maintain the fluid volume in the blood and intestines. Salt and soda, dissolved in water and sipped slowly so as not to cause vomiting, may be taken.

Replacement of potassium. Potassium regulates the intracellular osmolarity enzyme system, serves as a conductor of nerve impulses, and is necessary for the functional integrity of cells. It is not stored by the body; therefore daily intake is necessary. To replace potassium, the patient may ingest one 8-ounce glass of any of the following:

1. Tea or cola
2. Orange juice or tomato juice
3. Bouillon or consommé
4. Drinks developed for athletes (such as Gatorade)

It is important that the physician be aware of any symptoms of fluid loss and dehydration so that replacement amounts and types may be ordered.

CHAPTER 12

Nutritional considerations for the ostomate

In the early periods of civilization, living conditions were simple, and although the body's craving for food required satisfaction, there was little demand in the consideration of diet. Modern civilization's complicated mode of living, however, has seriously affected the body's energy-producing processes. Since many diseases are known to have been caused by improper diet and disturbed digestive processes, the proper quantity and quality of diet must be observed if the body is to maintain optimum nutritional status.

Nutrition is the combination of processes by which the living organism receives and utilizes the materials necessary for the maintenance of its functions and for the growth and renewal of its components. Normally, the sensations of hunger and thirst regulate the taking of nourishment. Hunger may be temporarily stilled by filling the stomach with indigestible substances, but the feeling soon returns, intensified, and can be allayed only by the ingestion of nutritive substances. The body's need for water is urgent. Living cells require water in order to function. Water is the basis of the body's blood and lymph system, which transports food and oxygen to the tissues and waste products from them. Water regulates the body temperature, and if the intake and output become imbalanced, kidney functions may be impaired.

Nutritional needs, likes, dislikes, and even appetites differ with the individual. ''What is food to one man may be fierce poison to others''* expresses a certain amount of truth, depending on the varying digestive powers of individuals. It is common knowledge that some foods have peculiar, almost poisonous effects on certain persons; the individual must discover these allergy-producing foods and learn to avoid them. Eating habits are personal and usually deep-rooted, since most of them are formed early in life, but they should be changed if food intake is not well balanced.

No one rule for the proper nutrition of all persons can be formulated, but on broad principles the best diet is one that contains nutrients vital to the growth

☐ Contributed in part by Jean N. Faulkner, R.D., Stouffer's Management Food Service, Tucson Medical Center.

*Lucretius, 98-55 B.C.

and maintenance of the human body. The human need for nutritional intake is based on stature, age, sex, and the expending of energy. Protein is essential for growth and repair of body tissue; carbohydrates and fats are necessary for energy; minerals and vitamins aid growth and prevent certain deficiency diseases; and water is important for all body functions (Chapter 11). The nutrient value of any food depends on its relative content of these components and on its caloric value (that is, the amount of energy generated when it is metabolized by the body).

Dietitians and nurses are aware of the need for special study in the science of nutrition as it applies to nourishing the individual in the hospital and in teaching the patient to manage his dietary needs after he has been discharged. The graduate nurse has some knowledge of diet therapy and, with the help of the dietitian, is able to incorporate this knowledge into daily nursing care plans. The patient's nutritional status is an important factor in his ability to survive the stresss of surgery, and physicians recognize that diet therapy is a vital element in total patient care.

The therapeutic diet is planned as a modification of the normal diet; every therapeutic diet should contain adequate amounts of the essential nutrients as defined in *Recommended Daily Allowance** (exceptions are specific nutrients ordered by the physician, depending on the patient's diagnosis). It is important that the dietitian, nurse, family, and physician work as a team in planning for the patient. Knowledge of the patient's eating habits, sex, age, weight, and activity level will guide the dietitian in planning a well-balanced diet. Children have greater needs for some nutrients because they are active and growing. The child's likes and dislikes should be considered if possible, since there are many substitute nutrients. The important factor is to provide the proper nourishment.

Elemental diets. Today, the inability to eat is seldom considered as an avoidable factor, since advances in nutrition have made it possible to supply the patient with complete nourishment through liquid preparations. There are commercial preparations on the market representing a different concept in nutritional feeding. These soluble powders, which provide a palatable solution, are of pure basic nutrients. Available in several flavors, these bulk-free total nourishment products may be consumed as a beverage or used as a tube feeding. They are composed of chemically discrete, readily absorbed, and rapidly assimilated nutrients—pure amino acids, vitamins and minerals, simple carbohydrates, and essential fat. The products require minimal digestion prior to absorption through the intestinal wall, have no indigestible matter, and reduce residue to that originating within the body itself. These chemically defined, bulk-free, elemental diets are recognized in the preoperative preparation and the postoperative management of the patient when the decompression

*Food and nutrition, National Academy of Sciences–National Research Council.

of the large gut is significant. The preparations may be taken into the body orally or through feeding tubes. Caution should be exercised when placing patients on sodium-restricted or elemental diets.

Feeding tubes. Solutions for tube feedings may be prepared in the diet kitchen or pharmacy. This type of feeding is especially beneficial to the immediate postoperative laryngectomee, who is not fed orally until tissues have healed, since damage or infection to the surgery area might ensue. Patients with pancreatic fistulas also benefit from this special nutritional preparation. It may be utilized in infant feedings when the establishment of bowel function is delayed following corrective digestive surgery.

The oral route is commonly recognized as the best course for satisfying nutrition requirements. Patients who are unable to swallow residue foods may be completely nourished orally by liquid preparations. However, this route is often prevented or precluded by disease or surgery, and feeding tubes placed through the nose or rectum or directly into the stomach are used. Biochemical monitoring is advised.

Special properly balanced hyperalimentation solutions, made by the hospital pharmacy and administered parenterally, offer the patient new opportunities to recover. Special precautions are necessary with this intravenous feeding, since the composition of this solution makes it a fertile medium for the growth of *Candida,* a genus of yeastlike fungi. The following precautions are suggested:

1. Only intravenous catheters, with the tip of the catheter inserted in the superior vena cava or inferior vena cava (not in the peripheral veins), should be used, since thrombosis may result if a high concentration of dextrose is given intravenously through the peripheral veins.
2. Use of aseptic technique is imperative. A minor preparation is necessary to avoid infection, and the attendent should wear sterile gloves.
3. All intravenous hyperalimentation solutions should be used within an hour after being constituted. If administration is delayed, the solution should be refrigerated immediately. Before this refrigerated solution is administered, the pharmacy should verify that it is still acceptable and present a method for bringing it to room temperature.
4. This intravenous set must have a special filter that, if properly used, will filter out most bacteria.
5. The tubing and filter should be changed every 24 hours. Aseptic technique must be used when loosening the tubing from the insertion site and when replacing the new tubing. The needle site should not be disturbed.
6. After removal, all filters should be sent to the microbiology laboratory for culturing.
7. If cloudiness or debris is noted in the solution or if cracks are seen in the bottle, the entire set should be removed and cultured.

The ostomate's new surgery does not alter individual eating habits once the stoma is well established (approximately 6 weeks). Preoperative intake is limited to fluids in order to decompress the small and large intestine, but postoperatively, intake increases slowly until a regular diet can be tolerated. Although the ostomate's diet depends on the individual and the surgery performed, an important factor to any ostomy patient, and particularly to the ileostomate, is that the fluids of the body remain in balance. Foods high in sodium and potassium are used in maintaining electrolyte balance, and a variety should be included in the diet.

The senses of taste and smell are reduced in the laryngectomee, since he no longer breathes through his nose. Although the senses will gradually improve, all foods will taste bland for a long period of time. Care should be exercised in making the diet nutritious and as attractive as possible to tempt the patient's appetite.

Ostomates as individuals have different digestive abilities and food preferences. It is essential that the dietitian plan meals with the patient until he is able to adjust to regularity. Diet should be discussed with each patient before discharge from the hospital. It is important that the ileostomate be cognizant of the sodium and potassium content of his intake to prevent electrolyte imbalance. Since some foods are indigestible or make the stool liquid, all foods should be introduced one by one until the patient learns which foods to avoid. The ostomate should keep in mind that foods that caused distress before surgery will cause distress after surgery. The following suggestions may aid in planning diets for the ostomate.

Low-residue diet. Residue is substance left in the large intestine after food is digested. A low-residue diet is often needed to maintain nutritional status in the ostomy patient. Hospitalized patients are usually placed on a low-residue diet to reduce bulk in the digestive tract. Low-residue foods are included in Table 2.

Table 2. Low-residue foods

Food	Included	Excluded
Beverages	Milk, limited to 1 pint (as such or in cooking), boiled if necessary	All other
	Coffee, tea, Postum	
Breads	Enriched toasted white bread, plain white crackers, Melba toast	All other
Cereals	Cooked cream of wheat, farina, cream of rice, cornmeal, hominy grits	
	Cooked strained oatmeal, pettijohns, other whole-grained cereals	
	Refined dry cereal such as puffed rice, puffed wheat, Rice Krispies, cornflakes	
	Rice, macaroni, spaghetti, noodles	All other

Continued.

Table 2. Low-residue foods—cont'd

Food	Included	Excluded
Desserts	Clear flavored gelatin and rennet desserts, custard, plain puddings, fruit whips (from allowed fruits), ice cream, sherbets, plain cakes, plain cookies	Nuts, coconut, raisins; rich pastries and desserts
Fats	Butter and margarine; cream in moderation	All other
Fruits	Bananas; canned peaches, pears, and applesauce; other fruits strained Strained fruit juices	Canned or fresh pineapple, berries, figs; raw fruits except bananas
Meats, egg, and cheeses	Tender beef, lamb, veal, chicken, turkey, liver, white fish, crisp bacon, tender lean roast pork, oysters, sweetbreads and brains, salmon, tuna Cream cheese, cottage cheese, mild cheddar cheese (combined with other foods) Eggs any way except fried	All cured and highly seasoned meats; any meat that has a tough fiber or gristle; fried foods
Soups	Any strained soup made from foods allowed	
Vegetables	All tender cooked asparagus, carrots, beets, young peas, young snap beans, spinach, squash White and sweet potatoes, without skins All other vegetables strained Tomato juice	All gaseous vegetables, raw or cooked, such as broccoli, brussels sprouts, cabbage, corn, turnips, cauliflower, cucumbers, green peppers, onions, radishes, and sauerkraut; all other raw vegetables; dried peas and beans
Miscellaneous	Salt and sugar in moderation Cream sauces, cocoa, jelly, honey, hard candy	Pepper, highly seasoned foods; pickles, relishes, jams, nuts, olives, popcorn, potato chips

Foods easily digested. Baked or mashed potatoes, refined rice, bouillon, cream soups, and macaroni or noodles are easily digested. Cheese may be added to foods for flavor. Vegetables should be well cooked and in some cases pureed.

Meats. Tender well-chewed meats are usually tolerated. Roasting, boiling, or broiling are the accepted cooking methods used by most ostomates in meat preparation.

Foods often avoided. Gas-producing foods cause discomfort and sometimes problems in social acceptance. The chief offenders are the cabbage family, mature beans, onions, cucumbers, and radishes. In addition to these foods, ostomates should avoid nuts, seeds, fried foods, whole-grain cereals, popcorn, rich spicy foods, corn on the cob, coconut, fresh celery, pineapple, and fresh grapes. Asparagus need not be avoided, but its odor is carried through the body and is noticed at the time of urine output.

Meals. Good food is to be enjoyed, but it is essential that meals be taken in a leisurely fashion at regular intervals and that snacks and ice cold drinks be cut to a minimum. Increasing the mastication of food is part of the new ostomate's instruction.

Prepared foods. Foods may be purchased packaged with proper nutrients or in special diets. Size of portions will vary, depending on the remaining digestive organs and the needs of the individual.

Foods containing sodium and potassium. See Table 3.

Table 3. Foods containing sodium and potassium*

	Portion	Grams	mg K+
Fruits			
Apricots, canned in syrup	3 medium halves	100	234
Apricots, dried, uncooked	6 halves	40	352
Apricots, raw	2 to 3 medium	100	281
Avocado, raw, pitted, peeled	¼ (3¼ × 4 inches)	50	302
Banana, raw, peeled	1 small 6-inch	100	370
Cantaloupe, raw	¼ (5-inch diam)	100	251
Grapefruit juice, fresh	½ cup	125	203
Grapefruit-orange juice, canned	½ cup	125	230
Honeydew melon, raw	¼ (5-inch diam)	100	251
Kumquats, raw	5 to 6 medium	100	236
Nectarines, raw	2	100	294
Orange, whole, peeled	1 small	100	200
Orange juice, canned	½ cup	125	249
Orange juice, fresh	½ cup	125	250
Orange juice, frozen concentrate, diluted	½ cup	125	233
Papaya, raw	⅓ medium	100	234
Peach, raw	1 medium	100	202
Peaches, canned in juice	2 medium halves, 2 Tbsp juice	100	205
Peaches, dried, uncooked	¼ cup	40	380
Plums, damson, raw	2 medium	100	299
Prunes, dried, cooked	5 medium, 2 Tbsp juice	100	327
Prunes, dried, uncooked	4 large	40	307
Prune juice, canned	½ cup	125	294
Raisins, dried, seedless	¼ cup	40	305
Tomato juice, canned	½ cup	125	264

*From Department of Food Services, Nutrition Services, University Hospital, Arizona Health Sciences Center, Tucson.

Continued.

Table 3. Foods containing sodium and potassium—cont'd

	Portion	Grams	mg K+
Vegetables			
Artichoke, cooked	1	100	301
Asparagus, frozen, cooked, drained	6 spears	100	220
Beans, baby lima, frozen	½ cup	85	335
Beans, kidney, canned, solids and liquids	½ cup	125	330
Beans, kidney, cooked	½ cup	125	425
Beans, lima, canned, drained	½ cup	115	255
Beans, lima, fresh cooked, drained	½ cup	85	359
Beans, pinto, cooked	½ cup	125	425
Beans, white, cooked	½ cup	100	416
Beets, cooked, drained	2 (2-inch diam)	100	208
Beet greens, cooked, drained	½ cup	73	242
Broccoli, fresh, cooked, drained	½ cup	77	206
Brussels sprouts, fresh, cooked, drained	½ cup (≈5)	76	205
Brussels sprouts, frozen, cooked, drained	½ cup (≈5)	76	214
Carrots, raw	1 large, 2 small	100	341
Chard, fresh, cooked	½ cup	83	266
Chard, raw	½ cup after cooking	83	457
Collards, fresh, cooked	½ cup	100	234
Collards, frozen, cooked	½ cup	100	236
Corn, frozen kernels on cob	1 medium ear	100	234
Dandelion greens, cooked	½ cup	100	232
Dandelion greens, raw	½ cup after cooking	100	397
Endive (leaves)	20 small; 40 long	100	294
Mushrooms, fresh	10 small; 4 large	100	414
Mustard greens, fresh, cooked	½ cup	100	220
Parsnips, fresh, cooked	½ cup	100	379
Peppers, green	1 large	100	213
Pickles, cucumber, dill	1 large	100	200
Potato chips	10 (2-inch diam)	20	226
Potatoes, french fried	10 (2 × ½ × ½-inch)	100	475
Potatoes, frozen, french fried	10 (2 × ½ × ½-inch)	57	372
Potatoes, fried from raw	½ cup	85	659
Potatoes, hashbrown	½ cup	100	475
Potatoes, white, baked in skin	1 medium	100	503
Potatoes, white, boiled with skin	1 medium	100	407
Potatoes, white, boiled without skin	1 medium	100	285
Potatoes, white, canned, solids and liquids	½ cup	125	250
Potatoes, white, mashed	½ cup	100	250
Pumpkin, canned	½ cup	115	276
Soybeans, cooked	½ cup	100	540
Spinach, boiled, drained	½ cup	90	324
Spinach, canned, drained	½ cup	90	227
Spinach, frozen, chopped, cooked, drained	½ cup	100	333

Table 3. Foods containing sodium and potassium—cont'd

	Portion	Grams	mg K+
Squash, winter, baked	½ cup	100	461
Squash, winter, boiled, mashed	½ cup	125	333
Squash, winter, frozen, cooked	½ cup	100	207
Sweet potatoes, baked in skin	1 small	100	300
Sweet potatoes, canned	1 small	100	200
Sweet potatoes, fresh, boiled in skin	1 small	100	243
Tomatoes, boiled	½ cup	100	287
Tomatoes, canned	½ cup	100	217
Tomatoes, ripe, raw,	1 small	100	244
Tomato juice, canned	½ cup	100	227
Turnip greens, canned, solids and liquids	½ cup	100	243
Vegetable juice cocktail	½ cup	125	276
Meats, fish, and poultry			
Bacon, Canadian, unheated	1 oz	30	111
Beef, average, for all cuts, raw	1 oz	30	101
Catfish, freshwater fillets, raw	1 oz	30	94
Cod, flesh only, raw	1 oz	30	108
Flounder, flesh only, raw	1 oz	30	97
Halibut, flesh only, raw	1 oz	30	127
Ham, cured lean	1 oz	30	97
Herring, flesh only, raw	1 oz	30	119
Ocean perch, Pacific, raw	1 oz	30	111
Salmon, pink, canned	1 oz	30	98
Sardines, canned in oil, drained	1 oz	30	137
Scallops, muscle only, raw	1 oz	30	112
Shad, flesh only, raw	1 oz	30	94
Sole, flesh only, raw	1 oz	30	97
Veal, average for all cuts without bone, raw	1 oz	30	91
Dairy products			
Buttermilk, from skim milk	1 cup	245	343
Milk, condensed, undiluted	½ cup	153	480
Milk, evaporated, undiluted	½ cup	126	382
Milk, low-fat, fluid	1 cup	246	431
Milk, nonfat, dry solids, instant	¼ cup	26	449
Milk, whole, fluid	1 cup	244	347
Skim milk, fluid	1 cup	245	355
Yogurt, from skim milk	1 cup	245	350
Yogurt, from whole milk	1 cup	245	323
Bread and bread products			
Bread, Boston brown	1 slice (3-inch diam × ½-inch)	35	104
Bread, pumpernickel	1 slice (4½ × 3½ × ⅜-inch)	32	145
Muffin, whole wheat	1 average slice	40	117
Pancake, buckwheat	1 average (4-inch diam)	45	110
Rice, Spanish	½ cup	75	174

Continued.

Table 3. Foods containing sodium and potassium—cont'd

	Portion	Grams	mg K+
Roll, whole wheat	1 average	35	102
Waffle, plain	1 (5½-inch diam)	75	109
Wheat germ	1 oz; 3 Tbsp	28	232
Miscellaneous			
Almonds, dry, salted	6 to 8	8	53
Bouillon, meat extract	1 cube	4	108
Candy, plain, milk chocolate	1 oz	30	109
Candy, semisweet	1 oz	30	92
Cashews	6 to 8	15	70
Catsup	1 Tbsp	17	62
Chili sauce, canned	3 Tbsp	50	185
Chocolate syrup	1 Tbsp	20	39
Coca cola	½ cup	113	59
Cocoa, average dry	1 Tbsp	7	98
Coconut, shredded	2 Tbsp	15	116
Coffee, instant, Nescafé	1 tsp	2	62
Coffee, roasted, Sanka, dry	1 tsp	2	40
Coffee, roasted, regular, dry	1 tsp	2	32
Curry powder	1 tsp	2	37
Lemon-lime soda	½ cup	113	38
Maple syrup	1 Tbsp	20	26
Mixed nuts	8 to 12	15	84
Molasses	1 Tbsp	20	300
Orange Crush soda	½ cup	113	113
Peanut butter	1 Tbsp	15	123
Peanuts, roasted	1 Tbsp	15	111
Pecans	12 halves; 2 Tbsp	15	63
Postum, dry	1 tsp	1	22
Sugar, brown	1 Tbsp	14	32
Walnuts, English or black	2 Tbsp	15	69

CHAPTER 13

Medications and treatments

Medicine, according to Hippocrates, is that which was invented for the sake of the sick; Herophilus (300 B.C.) termed medicine "the hands of the gods." In more modern terms we refer to medicine as the art or science of treating, curing, and preventing disease, relieving pain, and improving health.*

Old medical writings contained prescriptions for unusual mixtures such as a teaspoon of powdered acarus (mites) for fecal incontinence. To relieve obstruction, Hippocrates prescribed the drinking of the juice of spurge that had been poured into figs and allowed to ferment. He also advocated suppositories made of honey anointed with the gall of a bull to be inserted rectally two or three times, followed by an enema. Some medications in the sixteenth and seventeenth centuries were extremely dangerous to the patient, for example, the swallowing of large doses of crude mercury and bullets of lead or gold for the purpose of pushing an obstruction through the intestines.*

DRUG EFFECTS†

Today's increased knowledge, gained through scientific studies of the side effects and benefits of medications, has resulted in a more successful matching of medications to problem and patient. The ostomy patient, because of a decreased intestinal ability to handle medications, is particularly sensitive to toxic side effects.

Absorption of the drug product from the gastrointestinal tract is necessary for drug effect. Absorption is slower and less complete when the drug product is an enteric-coated tablet or a firmly compressed tablet. Drugs in the form of powders and liquids are more rapidly and completely absorbed. For some ostomy patients to receive the full benefit of medications, they may be required to chew the tablets or dissolve them in a liquid before swallowing.

Except in selected cases, pain medications are seldom required for more than a few days postoperatively. In instances in which pain persists and pain medications are necessary for longer periods of time, the ostomy patient should be aware that constipation may be a side effect of the drug. Laxatives

*From the history collection of Reba Grubb.

†Contributed by Jacqueline R. Womble, B.S., R.Ph.

or stool softeners (refer to Table 4) can be used to compensate for this side effect.

Antianxiety medications, frequently referred to as tranquilizers, may be of value until the patient rebuilds his strength, sleeps more normally, or becomes psychologically adjusted to a changed body image.

A wide variety of medications that do not require a physician's prescription is available to the ostomate via self-selection and purchase in supermarkets and convenience stores. Self-prescribing of nonprescription medications often results in adverse effects, and this can be a serious problem to the patient with a diversionary ostomy. Physicians and pharmacists are more aware of the need for caution in the choice of drug therapy and in dosage adjustments and should always be consulted *prior* to any medication changes.

Medications that are of particular application to ostomates and that have been successfully used by ostomates are presented in Table 4. Those drugs and comments about them are listed only as a guide to the individual needs of the patient. Tables 5 and 6 provide information regarding those medications that have the potential to cause a change in color of urine or feces.

Table 4. Topical and gastrointestinal drugs*

Medications	Action and use
Skin preparations	
1. Prednisolone aerosol (Meti-Derm) Triamcinolone spray (Kenalog, Aristocort) Nystatin cream (Mycostatin) Compound tincture of benzoin	1. Topical. To relieve irritation and itching. Nystatin is antifungal. Caution: Greasy base sprays and creams may interfere with appliance adherence.
2. Karaya powder Karaya paste	2. Topical. To protect reddened skin, to allow healing, and to increase adhesion of appliances.
3. Aluminum hydroxide suspension (Amphojel) Aluminum hydroxide and magnesium hydroxide suspension (Aludrox, Gelusil, Maalox, Mylanta)	3. Topical. For excoriated peristomal skin. The aluminum hydroxide in these products is the cooling, soothing ingredient.
Control of diarrhea	
1. Diphenoxylate (Lomotil) Paregoric	1. Oral tablet or liquid. To slow gastrointestinal motility.
2. Kaolin and pectin (Kaopectate) Bismuth subgallate (Devrom)	2. Oral suspension or tablet. To absorb excess fluid and aid in bulk formation.
3. Lactobacillus (Lactinex)	3. Oral tablet. To restore natural intestinal bacterial flora and aid in control of cold sores.
Control of odor	
1. Chlorophyll (Derifil)	1. Oral tablet. To deodorize feces; effectiveness is

*Courtesy Jacqueline R. Womble, B.S., R.Ph.

Table 4. Topical and gastrointestinal drugs—cont'd

Medications	Action and use
	questionable. May impart green-black color to fecal material.
2. Bismuth subgallate (Devrom)	2. Chewable tablet. To deodorize feces. May impart black color to fecal material.
3. Nil-Odor Banish	3. Appliance treatment. Place inside pouch to deodorize contents.
4. Acetylsalicylic acid (aspirin)	4. Appliance treatment. Place one 325 mg tablet inside pouch to deodorize contents. *Caution:* Do not let aspirin solution bathe stoma, as ulceration may occur.
Fecal softeners	
1. Dioctyl sodium sulfosuccinate (Colace) Dioctyl calcium sulfosuccinate (Surfak)	1. Oral capsule or syrup. To keep feces soft for easy, natural passage. Not a laxative; does not irritate the intestinal tract.
2. Psyllium hydrophilic mucilloid (Metamucil) Psyllium hydrocolloid (Effersyllium)	2. Oral regular or effervescent powder. To provide a smoothage effect to promote natural elimination.
Laxatives	
1. Bisacodyl (Dulcolax) Senna concentrate (Senokot) Danthron (Modane, tablet only)	1. Oral tablet or rectal (colostomy) suppository. Contact laxative action directly on large colon mucosa to produce peristalsis. Not active in small intestine.
2. Casanthranol with dioctyl sodium sulfosuccinate (Peri-Colace)	2. Oral capsule or syrup. Combines fecal softener (Colace) with a stimulant laxative (Peristim).
Casanthranol with dioctyl sodium sulfosuccinate and sodium carboxymethylcellulose (Dialose Plus)	Combines above (2) with water-retaining and lubricating properties.
Control of flatus	
1. Simethicone (Mylicon; also an ingredient in Kinesed, Mylanta, Di-Gel)	1. Oral tablet, chewable tablet, liquid. Defoaming action relieves flatulence by dispersing mucous gas pockets in gastrointestinal tract.

Table 5. Drugs that may discolor urine*

Drug	Color produced
Amitriptyline HCl (Elavil)	Blue-green
Cascara sagrada	Yellow to red
Chloroquine (Aralen)	Yellow to brown
Chlorzoxazone (Paraflex)	Orange to red
Danthron (Dorbane, Dialose Plus)	Pink to red

*Courtesy Jacqueline R. Womble, B.S. R.Ph.

Continued.

Table 5. Drugs that may discolor urine—cont'd

Drug	Color produced
Diphenylhydantoin (Dilantin)	Pink to red to red-brown
Ferrous salts (iron supplements)	Black
Furazolidone (Furoxone)	Rust-yellow to brown
Indomethacin (Indocin)	Green
Levodopa (Dopar, Larodopa, Sinemet)	Dark
Methocarbamol (Robaxin)	Dark on standing
Methyldopa (Aldomet)	Red to black on standing
Methylene blue	Blue-green
Metronidazole (Flagyl)	Dark
Nitrofurantoin (Furadantin)	Rust-yellow to brown
Phenacetin (in A.P.C. and Empirin)	Dark brown to black on standing
Phenazopyridine HCl (Pyridium)	Orange to red
Phenolphthalein (Agoral)	Red in alkaline urine
Phenolsulfonphthalein (PSP)	Red in alkaline urine
Phenothiazines (Thorazine)	Pink to red to red-brown
Phensuximide (Milontin)	Pink to red to red-brown
Quinacrine HCl (Atabrine)	Yellow
Quinine	Brown to black
Riboflavin (vitamin B_2)	Yellow
Rifampin (Rifadin, Rimactane)	Red-orange
Salicylazosulfapyridine (Azulfidine)	Orange-yellow in alkaline urine
Senna	Yellow to red
Sulfonamides (Gantrisin)	Rust-yellow to brown
Tolonium (Blutene)	Blue-green
Triamterene (Dyrenium)	Pale blue fluorescence
Warfarin sodium (Coumadin)	Orange

Table 6. Drugs that may discolor feces*

Drug	Color produced
Antacids	Whitish or speckling
Antibiotics, oral	Greenish gray
Anticoagulants	Pink to red to black†
Bismuth-containing preparations	Black
Charcoal	Black
Ferrous salts (iron supplement)	Black
Heparin	Pink to red to black†
Indomethacin (Indocin)	Green
Phenazopyridine (Pyridium)	Orange-red
Phenylbutazone (Butazolidin)	Pink to red to black†
Pyrvinium pamoate (Povan)	Red
Salicylates, especially aspirin	Pink to red to black†
Senna	Yellow

*Courtesy Jacqueline R. Womble, B.S., R.Ph.
†These colors may indicate intestinal bleeding.

CHEMOTHERAPY*

Chemotherapy is defined as the treatment of disease states by the administration of chemical agents. This terminology was first used for a class of antibiotics that were toxic to the disease organism but nontoxic to the patients. Chemotherapy more recently is equated with cancer chemotherapy. Cancer therapeutic agents are cytotoxic and must be administered with care. All other drugs employed in the treatment of disease are classified as pharmacologically therapeutic agents. Therapeutic agents include antibiotics, antihistamines, anti-infective agents, analgesics, antihypertensive agents, anti-inflammatory agents, and others. Therapeutic drugs, then, are classified as agents that act against a particular disease state or abnormality.

Cancer chemotherapeutic compounds are all very toxic agents because of their capacity to destroy rapidly reproducing cells. A relative balance between toxicity to cancer cells and to normal cells must always be considered. Rapidly reproducing normal cells that are most susceptible to toxic effects by cancer chemotherapeutic agents include (1) blood-forming elements, (2) mucosal cells of the gastrointestinal tract, and (3) skin and hair follicles. All patients receiving chemotherapy are observed carefully for these toxic effects. Ostomy patients, in particular, must be watched for stomal mucosal ulceration or bleeding, dehydration due to diarrhea, or obstructive constipation.

Chemotherapy may promote long remissions in cancer patients but in general is not curative.

RADIOTHERAPY†

Radiation therapy is often employed to destroy cancer cells and prevent spread both preoperatively and postoperatively. This therapy may also be used as a palliative measure for the comfort of patients with extensive malignancy. The theory of radiation therapy is not within the scope of this book. The concern here is that patients receiving therapeutic doses of radioactive isotope require modifications in the procedure of care. Procedures vary with the therapy used. The following procedure is suggested as a guide to the protection of personnel and visitors from excessive radiation when exposed to patients receiving 20 mc or more of radioactive isotope.

Supplies. The necessary supplies, other than two covered trash containers and four extra trash container linings and wire fasteners, are usually furnished by the Department of Nuclear Medicine. These include dosimeters, radioactivity signs, a radiation monitor, and urine and feces containers.

Orders. Usually the Department of Nuclear Medicine (DNM) routine orders will be incorporated into the physician's orders.

Personnel. Preferably only one nurse from each shift is assigned for patient care. The nurse must not be pregnant or have received cobalt or x-ray therapy. No other personnel are allowed in the room.

---

*Contributed by Jacqueline R. Womble, B.S., R.Ph.

†Contributed by Orpha Berrie, R.N., Head Nurse, Isolation Wing, Tucson Medical Center.

Preparation of patient before administration of radioisotope. Normal admission routine should be followed. To prevent unnecessary exposure, additional vital signs should not be checked after the patient is radioactive unless specifically ordered. If equipment is ordered, it should be left in the room in a designated place, usually on the wall behind the head of the patient's bed.

Before administration of the radioisotope, ambulatory patients should shower, and bed patients should be given a complete bath. To reduce radiation exposure of nurses, minimal patient care is given for the first 48 hours after the administration of the radioactive isotope.

The patient's gown or pajamas, robe, and slippers may become contaminated and need to be retained by the Department of Nuclear Medicine for 2 or 3 months before they are returned to the patient. The patient should wear a hospital gown. His slippers, robe, and pajamas should be disposable.

Preparation of room before administration of radioisotope. Two plastic-lined 30-gallon waste containers and extra liners should be placed in the room. One, labeled "Trash," is used for all disposable food containers. The other, labeled "Linen," is used for soiled linen and gowns that are not obviously contaminated. Ambulatory patients may remove filled bags for pick-up by the Department of Nuclear Medicine and replace the new bag.

The patient's valuable possessions should be removed from the room. Toilet articles and reading materials may be left in the room. The patient must be warned that these articles may become contaminated and must be held in storage for an extended time.

A plastic bag should be placed over the telephone receiver.

Procedures following administration of isotopes

Nursing personnel. Nurses should place signs on the door reading: "Radiation Area" and "No Visitors."

Dosimeters. Individual dosimeters with the name label of personnel caring for the patient must be worn on every shift. Dosimeters are read daily by the Department of Nuclear Medicine to monitor the amount of radiation.

Gowns, gloves, shoes. Gowns and gloves will be worn by personnel any time the room is entered for patient care and will be monitored before removal. If it is contaminated, the gown should be placed in a plastic bag. Gloves should be turned inside out and placed in the trash container. Since clothing may become contaminated by spills, personnel should wear old shoes and hose.

Patient unable to use bathroom or plumbing unsafe for radioactive isotope disposal. Radioiodine is excreted largely through the kidneys. If possible, the patient should void into a labeled container. If a bedpan is used, urine should be poured into a labeled container or down the toilet (only if the plumbing is safe).

For incontinent patients, an indwelling catheter is used and kept clamped, opened only at regular intervals.

Vomitus and feces are collected in a plastic bag, closed securely, and placed in a designated container. Paper feces specimen containers should be used for sputa. If any contaminated wastes are spilled, the nurse, wearing gloves, should wipe them up with paper towels or incontinent pads, place them in the waste container, and notify the Department of Nuclear Medicine immediately.

A room may be equipped with special plumbing. If the patient is in such a room, all wastes may be flushed down the toilet.

Dishes. Disposable isolation trays and dishes are used. Uneaten foods should be flushed down the toilet (if possible). Dishes and trays must be disposed of in the trash container.

Visitors. No visitors will be allowed for 48 hours after the isotope is administered, to limit unnecessary or dangerous exposure. After 48 hours, only visitors with specific permission from the attending physician may visit.

Visiting is limited to 2 hours a day, for each person, for the first week. Pregnant women, persons who have received x-ray or cobalt therapy, and children under age 18 are not allowed to visit.

Discharge of patient. After the patient is discharged, the Department of Nuclear Medicine will completely monitor the room before it can be cleaned. Any radioactive material will be removed by the Department via an outside door. The room cannot be released for occupancy until approved by the Department of Nuclear Medicine.

General references

Baran, R. B., and Rowles, B.: Factors affecting coloration of urine and feces, J. Am. Pharm. Assoc. **13:**139-142, March, 1973.

Block. L. H., and Lamy, P. P.: These drugs discolor the feces or urine, Am. Prof. Pharm. **34:** 27-29, Feb., 1968.

Dorland's medical dictionary, ed. 26, Philadelphia, 1976, W. B. Saunders Co.

Goodman, L., and Gilman, A.: The pharmacological basis of therapeutics, ed. 5, New York, 1975, The Macmillan Co.

Medical pharmacology, Lange Series, 1975.

Mercy Hospital, Rockville Centre, New York: Drugs and foods which may cause discoloration of the urine, Pharmacy Newsletter for Nurses **7:** March, 1973.

Physician's desk reference, ed. 30, Oradel, N.J., 1976, Medical Economics Co.

CHAPTER 14

The ostomy clinic, an extension of ostomy care

Ostomy services are an essential part of medical care, and the yearly increase in ostomy surgeries has focused attention on the urgency for meeting new requirements in this service. One way in which these requirements may be met is through the establishement of extramural or intramural clinics.

The extramural clinic, which may be community supported, subsidized by a nonprofit agency, or privately owned, provides a valuable service to the community. It would require a board of directors, a medical advisory staff, and personnel according to the scope of the program. The ostomy clinic within the hospital complex is probably the most useful on a general basis. It may be self-supporting, or the cost may be partially absorbed by the hospital services, since its direction would be regulated by the policies of the hospital's governing board. The hospital ostomy clinic may be either an entity within the department of nursing service or function as a division of the surgical and/or gastrointestinal medical services. In either case the ostomy nurse should be responsible for the management of the clinic and maintain a close contact with the nursing service department and the medical/surgical staff.

The clinic setting lends itself to all areas of ostomy care, and its services may be expanded to include related fields such as speech and occupational therapy, social services, nutrition, and restorative nursing. Large hospitals often lose contact with their patients after they are discharged; the clinic affords an opportunity for many interested professional specialists to meet, talk with the patient and his family, and employ the team concept of care, thus bridging the gap between hospital and home.

The preliminary step in establishing an ostomy clinic is to gain the enthusiastic support of a physician or physicians who can interest others in the project. The next step is to secure the approval of an administration that is committed to the clinic program and willing to supply the necessary equipment. Equally important is the endorsement of the medical/surgical staff of the hospital and the cooperation from the nursing service department. The medical team supervision and support should not be difficult to obtain, since medical professionals are cognizant of the fact that the concentration of ostomy cases in a special service can improve the care of the ostomy patient.

THE PLANNING COMMITTEE

A planning committee is selected, and its membership includes one or more interested physicians, the ostomy nurse, the director of nursing service, a member of the administration, a member of the finance department, and a qualified design consultant. It is the responsibility of this committee to:

1. Establish the objectives of the clinic
2. Conduct a survey of ostomy needs
3. Prepare a proposed program
4. Plan for adequate staffing
5. Arrange financing
6. Diagram the physical environment
7. Outline the operation of the clinic

Objectives

1. To meet the health and medical needs of the ostomy patient through a realistic program
2. To provide a specialized area where nursing personnel may have the opportunity to become more technically competent and skilled in ostomy care
3. To enhance the health status of the ostomy patient by providing continuity of care
4. To teach the patient precepts of healthful living as well as caring for his immediate problems
5. To coordinate activities with community agencies
6. To provide emergency service
7. To study and research new developments

Survey. To provide a realistic basis for planning, statistics reflecting the need for a clinic should be compiled from sources other than the hospital. A survey of the ostomy population in the hospital and surrounding locale should include the following:

1. The number of patients cared for in the hospital
2. The number of patients cared for in other hospitals in the community
3. The number of patients living in outlying areas
4. The care these patients are now being given
5. The estimated cost of this service
6. The availability of qualified personnel to staff the clinic
7. The potential for financing the clinic
8. The structural modifications that may be required to accommodate the program
9. The possibilities of coordinating transporation to and from the clinic for those unable to drive

Program. A functional program should reflect the uniqueness of the ostomy clinic. The immediate services should be matched with the demands as dictated by the information obtained through the survey. The scope of the ostomy program should include patients of all ages within and without the hospital domain. It should be broad enough to encompass all ostomy needs and flexible enough to administer aid at the time it is needed, since many of the ostomate's problems may be eliminated by prompt attention. For this reason an on-call coverage may be provided for both inpatients and outpatients. An answering service may be utilized after the clinic is closed and a telephone hot line for emergency situations.

Inpatient service. The clinic offers a setting conducive to teaching and coordination of discharge planning. The atmosphere approximates the home surroundings, and home care can be more realistically taught, without the distractions of a busy ward.

Outpatient service. These services will be important to:

1. The patient who is out of the hospital but still convalescing
2. The established ostomate who will return to the clinic for periodic stoma recalibration, skin problems, irrigation technique evaluation, and nutrition discussions
3. The potential ostomate who needs counseling

Staffing. The clinic will meet few of its objectives if it is poorly staffed. Greater efficiency will be attained by personnel selected for their ability in this field and their willingness to devote time to the clinic. An ostomy nurse or a registered nurse with special training should be the key member of the staff. An associate and a secretary or receptionist are basic staff requirements in the small clinic. The number of additional staff members will depend on the program of the clinic.

The responsibility of the staff should be clearly stated and the line of authority noted. The ostomy nurse should serve as a direct liaison between the clinic, administrative medical staff, nursing service, and other related departments and the community agencies who provide special services to the clinic clientele. The advisory committee should be comprised of a surgeon, a gastroenterologist, a urologist, an internist, and selected representatives from nursing service and related departments.

Financing the clinic. Clinics should, if possible, be self-supporting. However, service should not be refused if patients are financially indigent, nor should this specialized service penalize the patient who receives it. A well-planned clinic and teaching program will hasten a hospital discharge, thereby reducing cost to the patient.

It is not the purpose of this chapter to discuss fund-raising projects or to set patient charges. However, it would be expedient for those seriously considering a project to survey the community needs and the public resources and aids offered through various services supported by government or agency funds. These agencies are well aware of their service to the people and may have resources for such a project. Hospital and health insurance are also factors to be considered in the cost analysis.

The cost of service increases when the clinic is too complex to be efficiently staffed and utilized. Sometimes, to support itself, the price may far exceed the financial abilities of the average person, and those who require the service most will forego the need because of lack of finances.

Patient charges will depend on the service, the amount of financial support required to maintain the clinic, and the area served. When the nurse attends patients in other hospitals, in extended care facilities, or at home, travel charges should be made in addition to the patient charge.

Physical environment. Selecting the site for the clinic often determines the scope of its future usefulness. A professional consultant will be able to offer valuable advice concerning the site and design. Existing buildings should be explored before any decision is made about whether to redesign or build. The consultant will also be able to harmonize the ideas of the staff and mold them into an architecturally sound interior design. He will be knowledgeable of building codes and therefore have definite ideas on suitable materials, adequate heating, ventilation, lighting, and soundproofing. The following should be considered:

1. The design should reflect the purpose and facilitate the work of the staff.
2. The amount of space should be commensurate with the number of patients to be served.
3. The structure should not be so designed that it will soon become obsolete.
4. There should be a careful exploration of present needs, and an allowance for change or growth should be considered to prevent costly reconstruction later.
5. The clinic should be located close to the mainstream of medical care, where it can serve the acutely ill as well as the convalescent or the established ostomate.
6. There should be an outside entrance, easily accessible for outpatients.
7. Ventilation should be adequate and controlled to avoid drafts and maintained at a warm temperature.
8. Floors should be slip-resistant or carpeted.
9. Patients react positively to pleasant surroundings; therefore the interior should have an atmosphere of physical comfort and appeal.
10. Privacy, both visual and auditory, should be a prime consideration.

Space allotment. Efficient utilization of space within the clinic will provide areas for initiating the present program and allow room for expansion.

Reception area. The waiting room should be comfortable. Doorways should be wide enough to allow for the transportation of patients by wheelchair or stretcher.

Treatment room. This space should include:

1. Dressing area for the convenience of outpatients
2. Examining rooms or curtained cubicles

3. Stretcher with a foam pad, adjustable head, up-and-down elevation, and locked wheels (one for each examining room or cubicle)
4. Cabinets with sliding doors to contain all preparations, appliances, ostomy accessories, pillows, linens, bath blankets, towels, washcloths, cotton balls, plastic bags, and other pertinent supplies
5. Adjustable table for supplies
6. Wastebasket placed near the stretcher
7. Mirror

Bathroom. The bathroom should be well lighted and its arrangement comparable to the average home situation. Equipment needed would include:

1. Wall mirrors or an arrangement of mirrors to aid the patient in viewing the body areas while procedures are taught.
2. Light, portable tray table for equipment and supplies
3. Chair (commode height) placed near the commode
4. Standard or hook to hold the irrigation equipment
5. Stool (average height) for the instructor so that he is on eye level with the patient
6. A special shower stall (some patients prefer to use the shower stall for the irrigating procedure) with:
   a. Safety rails on the side walls
   b. Nonslip floor
   c. Soap dish high enough for the standing patient's convenience
   d. Shelf to hold supplies
   e. Two-way faucet with a hose (to wash the elimination from the shower floor)
   f. Conveniently located floor drain (essential for sanitation)
   g. Hooks to hold the irrigation equipment

Conference room. The conference area may be a space in the treatment room. If space is limited, conferences may be held in the ostomy nurse's private office or in the classroom area.

Staff space. The size of this area will depend on the number of staff members and their functions. In most cases two desks in the office will suffice.

Classroom. The classroom should be as large as the space will permit and should contain:

1. Table
2. Six to twenty chairs
3. Teaching supplies
   a. Educational materials for distribution to the patient or students
   b. Movie, overhead, and slide projectors
   c. Movie screen
   d. Cabinet to hold other teaching aids
4. Ostomy bookshelf (clinic staff members should be encouraged to keep current on new developments)

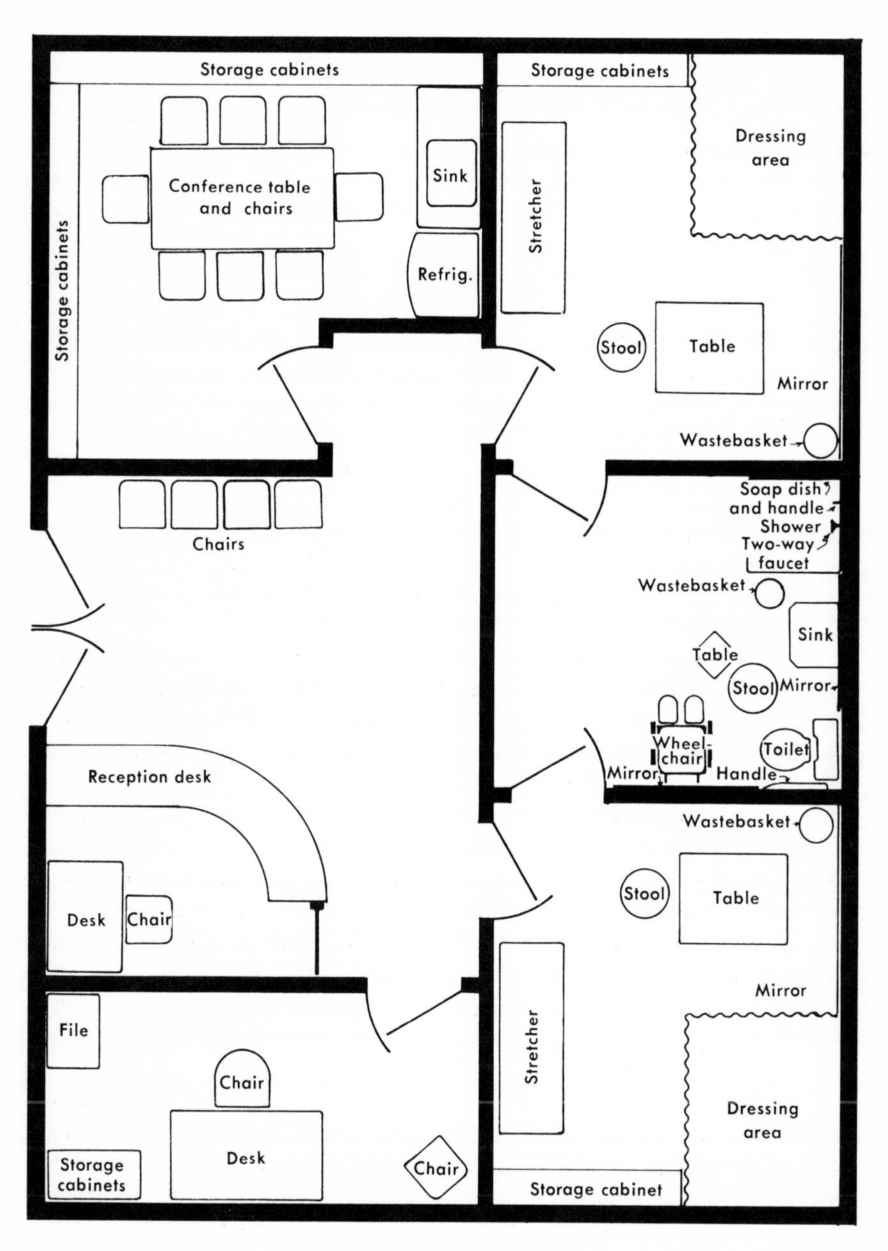

Fig. 14-1. Ostomy clinic layout.

a. Books and periodicals dealing with the various phases of ostomy care
b. Up-to-date reference list of related informational material that may be found in the hospital's library or other libraries in the community
c. Bibliographies compiled by the national and international associated agencies
d. List of ostomy chapters
e. List of surgical supply houses

Efficiency area. This small area may be included in the classroom design. There should be:

1. Refrigerator to hold juice or other liquids for use in patient care or teaching
2. Stove or hot plate for teaching simple diet preparations
3. Small cabinet for storing cups, pitchers, and dietary supplies

FACILITATING EFFICIENT CLINIC OPERATION

Manual. A manual of policies should be established and designed to accomplish the objectives, and procedures should be written to carry out the policies. The manual should be reviewed periodically and revised to incorporate any new developments in patient care. The policies should cover admissions, referrals, transfers, consultations, clinical services, charting, personnel regulations, and other pertinent information.

Records. Standardized forms should be adopted where possible to ensure continuity and understanding of the patient's care and progress. The patient's record is a continuous history, and the ostomy nurse should receive as much information as possible concerning the patient when he is referred to the clinic.

Reports and evaluations. Reports should be made either weekly or monthly to acquaint the hospital administration, nursing service director, administration, committees, or the community with the accomplishments of the clinic. Periodic evaluations should be made to assess and measure performance. A review committee may use these reports and evaluations to promote advancement in or expansion of the clinic. An annual report of progress should become a permanent part of the hospital's records.

SATELLITE CONTACT

A mobile ostomy service unit, complete with patient care facilities, equipment, and staff instruction aids is a valuable extension of the hospital clinic. It is a convenient method of providing direct contact with outlying communities and area hospitals.

In areas where an established clinic is not feasible, a mobile unit may serve as either a permanent or temporary clinic.

CHAPTER 15

Resources

Resources for the ostomy patient vary with locale; however, information is usually available through community health groups. Several services that may be utilized by the ostomy patient are listed here.

HOSPITAL SERVICES

A special services health team composed of representatives from various hospital services visits units in the hospital to offer consultation as needed. The team acts as an extension of other special services or as a liaison between special services and the physician, nursing services, or sometimes an extended care facility. The ostomy nurse is a member of this health team.

Restorative nursing. Restorative nursing focuses on rehabilitation. The restorative nurse is involved in helping the patient learn to live productively with diseases and disabilities, modifying patient and family attitudes of hopelessness concerning the disease while teaching them self-help.

Occupational therapy. In cases where the ostomy patient requires therapy, the occupational therapist performs a valuable service. Many of the diversions the patient learns in the hospital will assist him through his convalescence at home.

Physical therapy. The physical therapist serves as a consultant to the nurse regarding the patient's physical and functional needs. This service helps to develop special techniques to assist the patient in unusual situations (for example, the arthritic ostomy patient) or cord injuries that require ostomy surgery.

Speech therapy. The speech therapist is involved in the rehabilitation of the laryngectomee. Speech reeducation must be made after the surgeon decides that the muscles and mucous membranes are sufficiently healed to allow speech therapy. Artificial devices are available to help these patients, but most of them prefer to learn to speak with a "new voice" (esophageal speech) without devices. If a speech therapist is not available in the hospital, the surgeon or the social service department will be able to refer the patient to the proper resource.

Social service. Referrals to social services are approved by the physician, although the patient, his family, or nurse may request the referral. This service helps the patient and his family find solutions and make adjustments to interrelated physical, social, emotional, and economic problems and to receive the maximum benefit from medical care.

Therapeutic dietitian. The therapeutic dietitian helps the patient develop an understanding of the role diet plays in his new life. The dietitian serves as a consultant on basic nutrition and diet modification and helps the ostomy patient plan a normal diet from hospital to home.

Infection control. To prevent the ostomy patient from acquiring wound infections, the infection control service advocates aseptic technique and frequent hand washings as protective aids.

Auxiliary. The hospital auxiliary volunteers are trained to provide patients and their families with services tailored to cheer, educate, and support the need for personal attention. Volunteer activity in the health care field helps bring the hospital and community into a closer working relationship.

COMMUNITY RESOURCES

Visiting Nurse Association. The Visiting Nurse Association provides rehabilitative nursing care and treatment in the patient's home under the physician's direction and teaches a member of the family or household to give care between the nurse's visits. The Visiting Nurse sees the patient before he is discharged from the hospital and coordinates continued care at home using a nursing plan initiated at the hospital.

American Cancer Society. Aid and assistance are offered to the cancer patient, including information and referral to homemaker services, transportation, dressings, appliances, educational literature, and medication in indigent cases.

Assistance leagues and homemakers. Homemakers are available to provide supervised temporary assistance during emergencies. They are trained in allied medical health areas to care for the patient in the home.

Crippled Children's Association. This association provides assistance and diagnosis for children up to age 21 who are unable to afford private care. Eligibility provisions usually require that the patient be a resident of the state.

Veterans and military hospitals. Federal institutions recognize the needs of ostomy patients by either adding an ostomy staff nurse or securing consultations with appropriate specialists.

Extended care facilities and nursing homes. These facilities are available when permanent or temporary care for the ostomy patient's needs go beyond the acute hospital care.

Division of Vocational Rehabilitation. There are few jobs that cannot be filled satisfactorily by the ostomy patient who is well adjusted. If an ostomate requires further service to return to work, the division may be contacted and a plan of training for a new type of employment worked out. This is not a medically oriented service.

Medicare. All supplies for the ostomy patient eligible for Medicare are covered while the patient is hospitalized. The patient should receive ample supplies, enough to last for at least a week, 3 days prior to discharge to facilitate proper billing and eliminate additional expense for supplies after he arrives home. Clinical visits are a service to the patient, and therefore 80% will be covered by Medicare. Changes do occur in Medicare policies; a recent Social Security Act subsidized ostomy appliances for the outpatient. It is advisable for the patient to be aware of any current changes applicable to him. At this time, Medicare and Social Security do not cover services outside the United States.

Insurance. Insurance coverage generally includes all supplies necessary for the ostomy patient in the hospital. It is the responsibility of the patient to be aware of his individual policy and its benefits. Some permanent appliances and a supply of temporary pouches may be ordered 3 days prior to discharge.

United Ostomy Association, Inc. This is a needed service for new ostomates and their families. The group has continually grown in numbers as ostomy surgeries have become more numerous. Members of the group hold monthly meetings and include educational programs. This mutual aid group is especially helpful with information about appliances and manufacturers.*

Manufacturers of ostomy products. A partial listing of manufacturers is included in this resource chapter to guide the ostomate in securing the most suitable product for his individual needs.

Atlantic Surgical Company, Inc., 1834 Lansdowne Avenue, Merrick, L.I., New York 11566

Blanchard Ostomy Products, 2216 Chevy Oaks Circle, Glendale, California 91206

Coloplast/Bard, Inc., 731 Central Avenue, Murray Hill, New Jersey 07974

Davol Inc., Providence, Rhode Island 02901

Thomas Fazio Laboratories, P.O. Box 35, Assonet, Massachusetts 02702

John F. Greer Company, 5335 College Avenue, P.O. Box 2898, Oakland, California 94618

Gricks, Inc., 202-11 Jamaica Avenue, Hollis, New York 11423

Hollister Inc., 211 East Chicago Avenue, Chicago, Illinois 60611

Marlen Manufacturing and Development Company, 5150 Richmond Road, Bedford, Ohio 44146

Marsan Manufacturing Company, Inc., 5924 South Pulaski Road, Chicago, Illinois 60629.

Mason Laboratories, Inc., Willow Grove, Pennsylvania 19090

Nu-Hope Laboratories, Inc., 2900 Rowena Avenue, Los Angeles, California 90039

The Parthenon Company, 3311 West 2400 South, Salt Lake City, Utah 84119

Posey Company, 39 South Altadena Drive, Pasadena, California, 91107

E. R. Squibb and Sons, P.O. Box 4000, Princeton, New Jersey 08540

---

*Information may be obtained from the United Ostomy Association, Inc., 1111 Wilshire Blvd., Los Angeles, Calif. 90017.

Sween Corporation, Rapidan, Minnesota 56079
3M Company, Medical Products Division, St. Paul, Minnesota 55101
Torbot Company, 1185 Jefferson Boulevard, Warwick, Rhode Island 02886
United Surgical Corporation, Largo, Florida 33540

Artificial speech aids

Special Equipment Section, Commercial Department of local Bell Telephone Company Offices.
Aurex Corporation, 315 West Adams Street, Chicago, Illinois 60606
Brenkert and Deming, P.O. Box 47, Royal Oak, Michigan 48068
Rand Development Corporation, 12720 Lake Shore Boulevard, Cleveland, Ohio 44108

Special preparations—foods

Eaton Laboratories, Norwich, New York 13815
USV Pharmaceutical Corporation, Tuckahoe, New York 10707
Warren-Teed Pharmaceuticals Inc., Columbus, Ohio 43215

Suggested references

Alexander, N. B.: Towards independence with an ostomy, Queen's Nurs. J. **16:**250-251, Feb., 1974.

American Cancer Society: First aid for laryngectomees, International Association of Laryngectomees, 219 E. 42nd St., New York, N.Y. 10017.

American Cancer Society: A cancer source book for nurses, Boston, 1975, The Children's Hospital Medical Center.

Benson, H., and Klipper, M.: The relaxation response, New York, 1976, William Morrow & Co.

Berk, R., and Lasser, E.: Radiology of the ileocecal area, Philadelphia, 1975, W. B. Saunders Co.

Bevis, E.: Curriculum building in nursing, a process, St. Louis, 1973, The C. V. Mosby Co.

Bode, H., and Hendren, W. H.: Healing of fecal fistulas initiated by synthetic low-residue diet, Lancet **1:**954, 1970.

Bouchard, R., and Owens, N. F.: Nursing care of the cancer patient, ed. 2, St. Louis, 1972, The C. V. Mosby Co.

Brown, B.: New mind new body, Psychol. Today, Aug., 1974.

Cordonnier, J. J.: Simple cystectomy in the management of bladder carcinoma, Arch. Surg. **108:**190-191, 1974.

Cox, B., and Wentworth, A.: The ileal pouch procedure, Rochester, 1975, Mayo Comprehensive Cancer Center.

Creamer, B.: The small intestine, Chicago, 1974, Year Book Medical Publisher.

Davenport, H.: Physiology of the digestive tract, ed. 3, Chicago, 1971, Year Book Medical Publisher.

Davis, R.: Vesicoureteral reflex and Laura, Point of View (Ethicon) **9:**13-15, 1972.

Dericks, V.: The controversy over colostomy irrigation, Ostomy Quart., Spring, 1976.

Dericks, V.: Nursing care of patients with ostomies and pelvic exenterations, New York, 1974, American Cancer Society.

Detler, S. P., and others: Bilateral ureterostomy after ileal conduit diversion, J. Urol. **105:**365, 1971.

Dlin, B., Perilman, A., and Ringold, E.: Psychosexual response to ileostomy and colostomy, Am. J. Psychiat. **126:**374-381, 1969.

Dorland's illustrated medical dictionary, ed. 25, Philadelphia, 1975, W. B. Saunders Co.

Drach, G.: Diagnosis of urinary tract infection, Chicago, 1973, Kendall Hospital Products.

Dubay, E., and Grubb, R.: Infection: prevention and control, St. Louis, 1973, The C. V. Mosby Co.

Dudrick, S. J.: Minimizing sepsis risk in hyperalimentation. In The surgical team, Rowayton, Conn., 1976, McMahon Publishing Co.

Dworken, H. J.: The alimentary tract, Philadelphia, 1974, W. B. Saunders Co.

Ein, S. H., and others: Ulcerative colitis in children under one year: a twenty-year review, J. Pediat. Surg. **6:**264, 1971.

☐ Compiled by Martha Chrisman and Jean Good, Ostomy Education, Tucson Medical Center.

Enzel, G. L., and Morgan, W.: Interviewing the patient, Philadelphia, 1973, W. B. Saunders Co.
Epstein, C.: Nursing the dying patient, Reston, Va., 1975, Reston Publishing Co. Inc.
Ferguson, D. E. and Geist, R. W.: Pre-school urinary tract diversion for children with neurogenic bladder from myelomeningocele, J. Urol. **105:**133, 1971.
Gennaro, A. R., and Rosemouel, G.: Diverticulitis of colon, Dis. Colon Rectum **17:**74-81, Jan.-Feb., 1974.
Ghoneim, M. A., and others: Rectal bladder with perineal colostomy for urinary diversion, Urology **4:**278-281, Sept., 1974.
Gill, N., and Kerr, J.: Basic skin problems, Ostomy Quart., Spring, 1975.
Given, B., and Simmons, S.: Gastroenterology in clinical nursing, ed. 2, St. Louis, 1975, The C. V. Mosby Co.
Goldsmith, J.: Hobbies for patients: learning a skill is good medicine, Inservice Training and Education, June, 1973.
Grubb, R., and Blake, R.: Emotional trauma in ostomy patients, AORN J. **23:**52-55, Jan., 1976.
Grubb, R., and Mueller, J.: Designing hospital training programs, Springfield, 1975, Charles C Thomas, Publisher.
Gutowski, F.: Ostomy procedure: nursing care, Am. J. Nurs. **72:**262-267, 1972.
Haddad, J.: Colostomy treatment of traumatic injuries of the large intestines: a system of management, Dis. Colon Rectum **17:**188-193, March-April, 1974.
Jacobson, L.: Illness and human sexuality, Nurs. Outlook **22:**50-53, Jan., 1974.
Javett, S. L., and Brooke, B. N.: Reversed ileal segment for ileostomy diarrhea, Lancet **1:**291, 1971.
Jeter, K.: Count your blessings, New York, 1972, Columbia-Presbyterian Medical Center.
Jeter, K., and Bertsch, R.: Enterostomal therapy, better care for the ostomy patient, Am. Surg. **39:**124-126, Feb., 1973.
Jeter, K., and Bloom, S.: Management of stomal complications following ileal or colonic conduit operation in children, J. Urol. **106:**425, 1971.
Johnson, W.: Oral elemental diet: a new bowel preparation, Arch. Surg. **108:**32-34, 1974.
Jourard, S.: The transparent self, New York, 1971, Van Nostrand-Reinhold Co.
Klevins, C.: Materials and methods in adult education, New York, 1972, Klevens.
Knowles, M.: Modern practice of adult education, New York, 1971, New York Association Press.
Kramer, P., and Levitan, R.: Effect of 9-0 fluorohydrocortisone on the ileal excreta of ileostomized subjects, Gastroenterology **62:**235, 1972.
Kübler-Ross, E.: Death: the final stage of growth, Englewood Cliffs, N.J., 1975, Prentice-Hall, Inc.
Lapides, J., and Tank, E. S.: Urinary complications following abdominal perineal resection, Cancer **28:**230-235, 1971.
Lenneberg, E., and Rowbotham, J. L.: The ileostomy patient, Springfield, Ill., 1970, Charles C Thomas, Publisher.
Lysaught, J.: Instructional technology in medical education, Proceedings of Fifth Rochester Conference, Rochester, N.Y., 1971 Rochester Clearinghouse, University of Rochester.
Markgraf, W.: Mesh repair of abdominal wound dehiscence, AORN J. **22:**272, 274-275, 277-278, Aug., 1975.
McCaffery, M.: Nursing management of patient with pain, Philadelphia, 1972, J. B. Lippincott Co.
Media Horizons Staff: Video handbook, New York, 1974, Media Horizons, Inc.
Moser, S.: Social worker's role in ileostomy, AORN J. **23:**58-59, Jan., 1976.
O'Neill, J.: Ostomy for the neonate, training for the mother, Med. Surg. Rev., pp. 11-13, Aug.-Sept., 1971.
Orbach, C. E.: Ideas of contamination in postoperative colostomy patient, Psychoanal. Rev. **61:**269-282, Summer, 1974.

Peachy, R. D.: Proceedings: implantation of colonic mucosa in skin around colostomy, Br. J. Dermatol. **90:**108, Jan., 1974.

Perry, T. M., and Miller, F.: Pathology, Boston, 1971, Little, Brown and Co.

Physician's desk reference, ed. 30, Oradell, N.J., 1976, Medical Economics Co.

Popiel, E. S.: Nursing and the process of continuing education, St. Louis, 1973, The C. V. Mosby Co.

Ramirez, M.: Auditing of nursing care plans, Superv. Nurse **6:**29, 32, 34-35, June, 1975.

Sauer, G.: Manual of skin diseases, Philadelphia, 1973, J. B. Lippincott Co.

Schauder, M. R., and Joffrey, I. S.: Better management of fecal fistulae with stoma bags, R.N. **37:**56-57, May, 1974.

Schikedanz, H. R., and Mayhall, P.: Restorative nursing in a general hospital, Springfield, Ill., 1975, Charles C Thomas, Publisher.

Sparberg, M.: Ileostomy care, Springfield, Ill., 1971, Charles C Thomas, Publisher.

Spratt, J., Butcher, H., and Bricker, E.: Exenterative surgery of the pelvis. In Major problems in clinical surgery, Vol. XII, Philadelphia, 1973, W. B. Saunders Co.

Stroot, V., Lee, C., and Schaper, C.: Fluids and electrolytes, a practical approach, Philadelphia, 1974, F. A. Davis Co.

Tabers cyclopedic medical dictionary, Philadelphia, F. A. Davis Co.

Turnbull, R. B., Jr. and Weakley, F. L.: Atlas of intestinal stomas, St. Louis, 1967, The C. V. Mosby Co.

Wallace, G., and Hayter, J.: Karaya for chronic skin ulcers, Am. J. Nurs. **74:**1094-1098, 1974.

White, T., and Harrison, R.: Reoperative gastrointestinal surgery, Boston, 1973, Little, Brown & Co.

Williams, J.: Understanding the feelings of the dying, Nursing **6:**52-56, March, 1976.

Wright, H., and Tilson, M.: Postoperative disorders of the gastrointestinal tract, New York, 1973, Grune & Stratton, Inc.

Wyatt, J. K.: Ileal conduit diversion for benign disease, a critical review and long term follow-up, Can. J. Surg. **17:**270-273, Sept., 1974.

Sources for educational materials

American Management Association, Inc., The American Management Association Building, 135 W. 50th St., New York, N.Y. 10020.

Audiovisual Communications, United Business Publications, 750 Third Avenue, New York, N.Y. 10017.

Eaton Laboratories Publications, Division of Morton-Norwich Products, Inc., Norwich, N.Y., 13815.

Educational and Industrial Television, C. S. Tepfer Publishing Co., Inc. 607 Main St., Ridgefield, Conn. 06877.

Eli Lilly & Co., Medical Service Publications, Indianapolis, Ind.

E.T. Journal: official publication of the I.A.E.T.

Health Education Resources, Educational Management Associates, 20 N. Wacker Dr., Chicago, Ill. 60606.

Hollister, 211 E. Chicago Ave., Chicago, Ill. 60611 (ostomy publications).

Johnson and Johnson, New Brunswick, N.J. 08903.

Pfizer Laboratories, Division Educational Series.

Superintendent of Documents, U.S. Government Printing Office, Washington, D.C. 20401.

United Ostomy Association, Inc., 111 Wilshire Blvd., Los Angeles, Calif. 90017.

USV Pharmaceutical Corporation, Tuckahoe, N.Y. 10707.

The Vocational Guidance Quarterly, Business Office, 1607 New Hampshire Ave., N.W., Washington, D.C. 20009.

Warren-Teed Pharmaceuticals, Inc. Publications, Columbus, Ohio 43215.

Glossary

abdominal-perineal resection (AP resection) Surgical removal of the sigmoid colon, rectum, and anus and formation of a permanent colostomy.
abscess (L. *ab,* away or from, and *cedere,* to go) Localized collection of pus formed by the disintegration of tissues.
adhesion (L. *adhaerere,* to stick) Abnormal binding of parts to one another by a fibrous band.
albumin (L. *albus,* white) Term applied to a class of protein substances, some form of which is the essential part of every living cell.
alimentary canal (Gr. *alo,* to nourish) Entire tubular structure that extends from the mouth to the anus through which nourishment passes. It functions in the digestion of nourishment and the elimination of waste.
alkali (Ar. *al,* definite article, and *kali,* the plant from which soda was first obtained) Substance that reacts with acids to form salts.
ampulla of Vater (L. *amphora,* jar, and Vater for Abraham Vater, anatomist [1684-1751]) Flasklike passageway through which digestive juices empty into the duodenum.
amylase (Gr. *amylon,* starch) Enzyme that converts starch into glucose.
anastomosis (Gr. *ana,* through, and *stoma,* a mouth) Surgical joining together of two or more hollow organs, such as the joining of two loops of bowel after removal of a segment.
anterior (L. *ante,* before) Situated in front of; forward part of; ventral or belly surface of the body. Opposite of posterior.
anus (L. *annus,* a circle) End of the alimentary canal.
ascending colon (L. *ascendo,* to climb) First part of the large intestine, extending from the cecum to the right colic flexure.
barium (Gr., heavy) **sulfate** White chalklike substance used to outline the digestive tract for x-ray examination.
benign Not malignant.
biopsy (Gr. *bio,* life, and *opis,* vision) Excision of small piece of tissue or other material from the living body for microscopic examination.
casein (L. *caseus,* cheese) Principle protein of milk; basis of cheese and curd.
cecostomy Surgical creation of an opening into the cecum, usually only temporary; used to remove pressure in the large bowel.
cecum (L. *caecum,* blind) First portion of the large intestine; a blind pouch or cul-de-sac with openings from the ileum and appendix.
cellulose (L. *cellula,* a little cell) Substance that forms most of the framework of vegetable tissue.
chemotherapy (Gr. *chemeia,* chemistry) Treatment of disease by chemical agents.
choledochostomy (Gr. *chole,* bile, *dochos,* duct, and *ostomy,* opening) Surgical formation of an opening into the common bile duct.
chyle (Gr. *chulos,* juice) Thin milky fluid produced by intestinal digestion.

☐ To further define any term used, refer to a current medical dictionary.

chyme (Gr. *chumos,* juice) Partly digested semifluid contents of the stomach as they enter the intestine.
colitis Inflammation of the colon.
colon (Gr. *kolon*) Large intestine; begins in the right abdomen and extends from the cecum to the rectum.
colostomy Surgical creation of new opening in the colon.
congenital (L. *congenitus,* born together) Present at birth.
decompression Removal of pressure, as from gas in the intestinal tract.
decubitus (L., a lying down) Act of lying down; ulcer or bedsore.
deglutition (L. *de,* from, and *glutire,* to swallow) Act of swallowing.
dehiscence (L. *dehiscere,* to gape) Separation of all layers of incision or wound.
dehydration (L. *de,* from, and Gr. *hydor,* water) Condition resulting from excessive loss of water.
descending colon (L. *descendo,* to move downward) Part of the large intestine between the left colic flexure and the sigmoid colon.
diaphragm (Gr. *dia,* through, and *phragnunci,* to fence) Large muscle separating the thorax and abdomen; the midriff.
dilate Distend or stretch beyond normal dimensions.
distal (L. *distans,* distant) Farthest away from the beginning or central point.
diversion (L. *divertere,* turn aside) Variation or departure from the natural conditions.
diverticulum Little sac or outpouching in the walls of a canal or organ.
duodenum (L. *duodeni,* twelve) Division of the small intestine, so named because its length is equal to breadth of twelve fingers; the first part of the small intestine that connects proximally with the pylorus and extends to the jejunum.
dyspepsia (Gr. *dus,* ill, and *peptein,* to cook or digest) Imperfect digestion.
electrolytes Solutions of positive and negative ions capable of transmitting electricity.
endoscopy (Gr. *endon,* within) Procedure to visualize any cavity of the body by use of a flexible instrument, an endoscope.
enteritis Inflammation of the intestine, particularly of mucous and submucous tissues; usually refers to inflammation of the small intestine.
epidermis (Gr. *epi,* upon, and *derma,* skin) Thin insensitive layer of cells on the outside of the skin.
epithelium (Gr. *epi,* upon, and *thele,* nipple) Cells that cover the internal and external surfaces of the body, including the lining of vessels and other small cavities. It serves as a protection for the body and aids in secretion and absorption.
esophageal speech System of swallowing and expelling air through the mouth from the esophagus taught to laryngectomees so that they can speak again.
esophagus Tube connecting the mouth with the stomach.
excoriation (L. *ex,* from, and *corium,* skin) Red, raw skin; any superficial erosions and ulcerations produced mechanically.
excrement Waste matter discharged from the bowels; feces.
excretion (L. *ex,* out, and *cretus,* sifted) Elimination of waste products from the body.
exenteration (L. *ex,* out, and *entero,* intestine) Radical surgical procedure for excision of the contents of a body cavity.
exteriorize (L. *externus,* outside) Exposure of an organ or part that is brought outside the body cavity.
exudate (L. *exsudare,* to sweat out) Fluid or semifluid oozed through tissues into a cavity or on the body surface.
feces (L. *faex,* refuse) Excrement discharged from the intestines.
ferment (L. *fervimentum,* to leaven; boiling) To decompose; a substance producing chemical change in another substance without losing its own identity; for example, yeast liberates bubbles of gas.

fissure (L. *fissura,* to cleave) Painful slit or defect in the skin, often crusted.
fistula (L., pipe) Abnormal hollow passage from an abscess, cavity, or hollow organ to the skin or between two internal organs.
fundus (L., base or bottom base) Bottom of an organ or part of a hollow organ farthest from its mouth.
gall (Gr. *gaster,* stomach or pertaining to the stomach) Bitter secretion from the liver, stored in the gallbladder.
gastrointestinal series Series of diagnostic tests.
granulations (L. *granum,* a grain or grains) Grainlike bodies made up of large, soft vegetative cells that form on the surface of wounds and ulcers.
haustra (L., recess) Pouches or sacculations in the wall of the large intestine caused by the adaptation of the length of the intestines to the taenia coli.
ileum (L. *eilio,* to twist) Lower third division of the small intestine, so called because of its numerous coils or convolutions.
imperforate (L. *in,* not, and *perforere,* to bore through) Without an opening; abnormally closed.
impotent (L. *in,* not, and *possum,* to be able) Weakness; want of power, especially of virile power, incapable of procreating or impregnating.
incontinence (L. *in,* and *contineo,* to contain) Inability to control the natural evacuations.
inflammation (L. *in,* and *flamma,* flame) Tissue reaction to injury: redness, swelling, pain, increased heat.
intestine
large Colon.
small Elongated tube measuring up to 22 feet in length in the adult, lying proximal to the large intestine.
intravenous pyelogram (IVP) (within a vein; Gr. *pyelos,* pelvis, and *gramma,* mark) Visualization of the bladder and kidney through the aid of a dye injected into the vein.
ion (Gr., going) Atom or a group of atoms having a charge of positive (cation) or negative (anion) electricity.
jejunostomy Surgical creation of an opening through the abdominal wall into the jejunum.
jejunum (L. *jejunus,* empty) Second division of the small intestine extending from the duodenum to the ileum.
karaya Gum from the bark of a tree of India used as an accessory product in ostomy care.
laryngoscope Instrument used to examine the larynx.
laryngostomy Establishment of a permanent opening through the neck into the larynx.
larynx (Gr. *larugx*) Upper part of the trachea or windpipe; the organ of the voice.
lipase (Gr. *lipos,* fat, and pepsin) Enzyme that digests fats.
malignant (L. *malus,* evil) Applied to diseases that endanger life; tending to become progressively worse and to result in death.
mastication (L. *masticare,* to chew) Grinding the food with the teeth.
membrane (L. *membrana,* skin) Thin layer of tissue that covers a surface or divides a space or organ.
meninges (Gr., membrane) Three membranes that envelop the brain and spinal cord.
mesentery (Gr. *mesos,* middle, and *enteron,* intestine) Membranous fold attaching various organs to the body wall.
metastasis (Gr., to transpose) Invasive process of malignancy.
mucous membrane Lining of cavities and canals that communicate with external air.
mucus Fluid secreted from cells or glands that moistens the membrane.
myelomeningocele (spina bifida) (Gr. *myelo,* marrow, *meninges,* membrane, and *kele,* hernia or swelling) Protrusion of a portion of the spinal cord and membranes through a defect in the spinal column.
nasogastric (L. *nasalis,* pertaining to the nose, and *gastric,* stomach)

neoplasm (Gr. *neo,* new, and *plasma,* to form) New and abnormal growth.
nephrostomy Creation of a permanent fistula leading directly into the pelvis of the kidney.
neurogenic (Gr. *neuron,* nerve, and *genus,* origin) Originating in nerve tissue.
nuclear Pertaining to a nucleus; a general term used to designate a group of nerve cells ordinarily located within the central nervous system and bearing a direct relation to the fibers of a particular nerve.
omentum (L., coverlet) Fatty apron in front of the intestine.
orifice (L. *os,* mouth, and *facio,* to make) Mouth or entrance to any cavity of the body.
palliative (Gr., to hide or cloak) Affording relief but not cure.
pancreas (Gr. *pan,* all, and *kreas,* flesh) Gland about 1 inch in diameter and 6 to 8 inches long lying behind the stomach. It secretes a thin watery liquid called pancreatic juice, which is poured into the duodenum.
Papanicolaou smear (Pap smear) Method of staining smears of various body secretions for detection of malignant process.
patent (L. *patens,* to be open) Open.
pepsin (Gr. *pepsis,* to cook or digest) Lifeless ferment found in the stomach; digests albumin.
peptone (Gr. *pepton,* digesting) Secondary protein derivative of albumin.
perianal (Gr. *peri,* about, and *anus,* circle) Around or near the anus.
perineal Relating to the perineum.
perineum Space between the anus and the genital organs.
peritoneum (Gr. *peri,* about, and *teino,* I stretch) Very smooth serous membrane, the largest and most important in the body.
peritonitis Inflammation of the abdominal lining (peritoneum).
perspiration (L. *per,* through, and *spirare,* to breathe) Water secretion of the skin; sweat.
polyposis (Gr., many) Multiple polyps throughout the large bowel that sometimes develop into cancer; thought to be familial.
posterior (L. *posterus,* behind) Situated in back of or in back part of; back of the body.
proximal (L. *proximus,* next) Nearest the point of attachment or origin; opposite of distal.
purulent Consisting of pus; of the nature of pus.
pylorus (Gr. *pulouros,* gate-keeper) Orifice in right end of the stomach through which food passes into the intestine.
rectum (L. *rectus,* straight) Last, nearly straight, portion of the large intestine, terminating at the anus.
resection (L. *resectio,* to cut off) Surgical removal of a section or segment of an organ.
sacculations (L., little sac) Small sacs or pouches.
saliva Fluid secreted by the salivary glands to aid in mastication.
serous membrane Membrane lining a cavity that is not exposed to the air.
sigmoid (Gr. *sigma* Σ) Portion of the large intestine between the descending colon and the rectum, so named because it resembles the Greek letter sigma; curved like the letter S.
sphincter (Gr., bind tight) Circular muscle that contracts the aperture to which it is attached.
spina bifida; see **myelomeningocele**
stenosis (Gr., to make narrow) Constriction or narrowing of a passageway or opening.
taeniae coli (Gr. *taenia,* riband, and *coli,* colon) Three bands that run for 6 feet from the cecum to the rectum; ligaments of the colon, longitudinal muscular fibers gathered into three bands, shorter than the portion of the bowel to which they are applied and causing a shirring of the large intestine from the cecum to the rectum.
therapist (Gr. *therapeutes,* one who attends the sick) Person skilled in the treatment of disease; often combined with a term indicating the specific type of disorder treated.
trachea (L. *trachia,* windpipe; Gr. *trachys,* rough) Straight flexible tube that lies in front of the esophagus and extends from the larynx. It divides into two tubes known as the bronchi.
transverse colon (L. *trans,* across, and *verto,* to turn or direct) Portion of the colon that crosses the middle line below the stomach to the descending colon.

trauma Injury.
trypsin (Gr. *tryein,* to rub, and *pepsin*) Ferment of pancreatic juice that digests albumin.
ulcer (L. *ulcus*) Open sore on the skin or mucous membrane characterized by the disintegration of the tissue.
ulcerative colitis Inflammation of the colon that is acute or chronic in nature and associated remissions and exacerbations.
umbilicus Navel.
ureter Tube leading from the kidney to the bladder.
ureterostomy Formation of a permanent opening for ureters into the patient's abdomen so that the ureter may discharge its contents.
vagus nerve (L. *vagus,* wandering) One of the pairs of cranial nerves, also called the pneumogastric nerve, which supplies a sensory branch to the ear and motor branches to the larynx and pharynx. It then passes into the thorax and gives off branches to the heart, which restrain its action. It gives sensory branches to the esophagus and lungs and finally reaches the stomach and liver. The main nerve supply of these organs is from the spinal cord, or from the sympathetic system, but the vagus nerve is an additional means for better regulating their action to suit the needs of the body.
valvulae conniventes (L. *valvulae,* little sliding doors, and *conniventes,* winking; closing valves) Folds in the small intestine that prevent food from passing through the intestine too quickly and present a greater surface for the absorption of the digested food.
vesicotomy Incision of the urinary bladder.
villi (L. *villus,* shaggy hair) Fingerlike projections on the surface of the valvulae conniventes.
viscera Inner parts of the body, especially the abdomen.

Index